INTERPRETATION OF BLADDER BIOPSIES

Biopsy Interpretation Series

Biopsy Interpretation Series

Series Editor: Ancel Blaustein, M.D.

Biopsy Diagnosis of the Digestive Tract
Heidrun Rotterdam and Sheldon C. Sommers, 1981, 490 pages

Interpretation of Biopsy of Endometrium
Ancel Blaustein, 1980, 208 pages

Interpretation of Bladder Biopsies
Peter N. Brawn, 1984, 224 pages

Interpretation of Liver Biopsies
Richard J. Stenger, 1983, 176 pages

Interpretation of Prostate Biopsies
Peter N. Brawn, 1983, 144 pages

Melanoma: Histological Diagnosis and Prognosis
Vincent J. McGovern, 1982, 204 pages

Volumes in Preparation:

Interpretation of Biopsies of Soft Tissue Tumors
Artemis Nash

Interpretation of Breast Biopsies
Darryl Carter

Biopsy Interpretation of Diseases of Muscle
Alfred J. Spiro

Interpretation of Bladder Biopsies

Biopsy Interpretation Series

Peter N. Brawn, M.D.
Department of Surgical Pathology
St. Luke's Episcopal Hospital
Texas Medical Center
Houston, Texas

Raven Press ■ New York

Raven Press, 1140 Avenue of the Americas, New York, New York 10036

Made in the United States of America

Library of Congress Cataloging in Publication Data

Brawn, Peter N.
  Interpretation of bladder biopsies.

  (Biopsy interpretation series)
  Includes bibliographical references and index.
  1. Bladder—Tumors—Diagnosis. 2. Bladder—Biopsy,
Needle. 3. Diagnosis, Cytologic. 4. Bladder—Diseases—
Diagnosis. I. Title. II. Series.
RC280.B5B73   1984   616.6'20758   83-21320
ISBN 0-89004-258-6

Preface

The bladder, with the use of cystoscopy, is one of the most accessible internal organs to study. However, the histopathology of the bladder, to a large extent, has remained a mystery. There continues to be great controversy concerning such basic concepts as what represents malignancy of the bladder (papillomas versus papillary carcinomas) and concerning the origin of invasive bladder carcinoma (papillary lesions versus "flat" lesions). This controversy has caused difficulty in evaluating the results of various forms of therapy and in comparing mortality, survival, and other data.

In large part due to the work of Meyer Melicow and Leopold Koss, we are beginning to arrive at general concepts concerning the histopathology of the bladder. These concepts appear to be the basis on which further advances will depend. However, after innumerable years of controversy, it may be difficult for physicians to appreciate the true nature of neoplasia of the bladder.

This monograph is directed toward pathologists and urologists, in practice and in training, and is intended to provide a unifying theme concerning neoplasia of the bladder. The various chapters include normal histology, developmental abnormalities, inflammation, hyperplasia, papillary lesions of the bladder, carcinoma *in situ*, cytology, and miscellaneous malignant and nonmalignant lesions of the bladder. Each chapter is followed by a large number of photomicrographs.

Peter N. Brawn, M.D.

Acknowledgments

I thank Arch Brown, Wayne Eaton, Robert Fredenburgh, and George Greidenger of St. Joseph Hospital, Flint, Michigan, for providing material for the photomicrographs on cytology of the bladder.

I thank Michelle Fornier Smith, McLaren General Hospital, Flint, Michigan, and Dr. Mattie Bossart and Tin Tin Middleditch of St. Luke's Episcopal Hospital, Houston, Texas, for technical photographic supervision.

To my brother, R. James Brawn, M.D.

Contents

Chapter 1

Normal Histology

ANATOMY

The bladder is an expandable baglike structure, situated mainly in the pelvic cavity, but when expanded, it extends upward into the abdomen. The anterior wall of the bladder partially fuses with the anterior pelvic wall. The posterior wall is adjacent to the rectum in males and adjacent to the uterus and vagina in females.

The internal surface of the bladder contains a trigone located near the base of the bladder. This trigone is a triangular area bordered by two ureters and the internal urethral orifice. Opposite the trigone is the dome of the bladder, which represents the superior aspect of the bladder. Between the dome and the base are found the right and left lateral walls, the anterior wall, and the posterior wall.

HISTOLOGY

The bladder wall consists of mucosa, lamina propria, muscular wall, and serosa. The mucosa is termed "transitional epithelium" or, preferably, "urothelium." Beneath the mucosa is a loose area of connective tissue termed "lamina propria," which contains vascular and lymphatic channels. The major thickness of the bladder is accounted for by three layers of muscular tissue. These three layers cannot be readily distinguished from one another. Their respective thickness varies in different parts of the bladder. Part of the bladder is covered with peritoneum forming a serosa. The remainder of the bladder blends into adjacent connective tissue.

Urothelium

The bladder accommodates varying amounts of urine while maintaining a urine-blood barrier. The urine-blood barrier is largely maintained by a specialized epithelium. The bladder epithelium, or urothelium, a term coined by Meyer Melicow (1) in 1945, varies in thickness depending on the distention of the bladder. The urothelium normally varies from five to seven cells in thickness (Figs. 1.1 to 1.8). Larger superficial cells cover, in an umbrella fashion, smaller underlying cells. The superficial umbrella cells are often binucleated or multinucleated and vary in size and configuration depending on the degree of bladder distention. The superficial cells are flat and thin in distended bladders but become more cuboidal in contracted bladders. Superficial cells are easily shed and frequently lost in routine biopsy material. When present, the superficial cells are an indication of the relative normalcy of the urothelium. However, the presence of superficial umbrella cells is not

1

an infallible indication of normalcy since the underlying cells may be sufficiently atypical to warrant a diagnosis of atypia/dysplasia or, occasionally, carcinoma *in situ*.

Bladder Neck

The bladder neck has surface foldings and undulations that may be confused with a papillary tumor. These normal foldings of the bladder neck (Figs. 1.9 to 1.14) can usually be distinguished from papillary tumors by the presence of urothelium of normal thickness surrounding thick fibrous stalks. Furthermore, the bladder neck foldings may have an irregular appearance but rarely have an exophytic appearance.

Periurethral ducts (Figs. 1.15 to 1.18) adjacent to the bladder neck may be crowded and have a complicated appearance with areas of transitional metaplasia. These glands may be confused with either prostate carcinoma or an invasive lesion originating in the overlying urothelium.

PROLIFERATIVE LESIONS

Brunn's Nests

Brunn's nests (Figs. 1.19 to 1.24) are clusters of cells lying in the lamina propria adjacent to or in direct continuity with the urothelium. The clusters are composed of urothelial cells that are either solid or contain a suggestion of a central lumen. As the central lumen increases in size, the lesions are termed "cystitis cystica" or "cystitis glandularis." There appears to be a transition between Brunn's nests with a lumen and cystitis cystica and cystitis glandularis.

Brunn's nests are most commonly observed in the trigone or adjacent to the bladder neck but may be seen elsewhere in the bladder. Characteristic gross or cystoscopic findings are usually absent.

Cystitis Glandularis and Cystitis Cystica

Cystitis glandularis (Figs. 1.25 to 1.28) are urothelial cysts in the lamina propria lined by columnar cells whereas cystitis cystica (Figs. 1.29 to 1.36) are urothelial cysts in the lamina propria lined by simple stratified urothelium. These cysts may be associated with inflammation but are just as likely to be free of inflammation. The cysts range from 1 mm to several millimeters in diameter. Many observers have speculated that cystitis glandularis and cystitis cystica develop from cavitation of Brunn's nests.

In extreme cases, the presence of numerous and large cysts causes a characteristic cystoscopic appearance of "cobblestone" urothelium due to elevations caused by the cysts. Redness of the urothelium is sometimes recorded. However, in the majority of cases, cystoscopic findings are absent.

The cysts are usually confined to the lamina propria. Cysts occurring within the muscularis raise the possibility of the presence of an adenocarcinoma.

Significance of Proliferative Lesions

The presence of Brunn's nests, cystitis cystica, and cystitis glandularis in the lamina propria of the bladder has traditionally been considered to be abnormal. These proliferative lesions have usually been attributed to inflammation, metaplasia, or unknown proliferative stimuli.

The relationship between these proliferative lesions and the development of bladder carcinoma has been widely debated. There have been case reports of occasional associations of cystitis glandularis or cystitis cystica with bladder carcinoma (2). Furthermore, Brunn's nests may occasionally be the site of carcinoma *in situ*. However, L. G. Koss (3) has convincingly argued that these proliferative lesions may be interpreted as reflecting the spectrum of normal variants of bladder epithelium. Koss studied 100 grossly normal urinary bladders obtained at postmortem examination. There were 61 males and 39 females in the study. Ninety-two patients were 30 years of age or older, six patients were between the age of 10 and 20, and two were children younger than 1 year of age. In each bladder, 15 blocks of epithelium and of the underlying tissue were obtained. Ninety-two of the 100 bladders contained one or more of the proliferative lesions, i.e., Brunn's nests in 89 of the 100 bladders and cystitis cystica in 60 of the 100 bladders. Had more sections been taken, it is likely that proliferative lesions would have been found in all 100 bladders. Other studies (4) have shown no correlation between the presence of Brunn's nests or cystitis cystica and the presence of infection, stones, or catheters. Consequently, it appears that these proliferative lesions are not an indication of premalignant change but rather a normal variant of bladder urothelium.

REFERENCES

1. Melicow, M. (1945): Tumors of the urinary drainage tract: urothelial tumors. *J. Urol.*, :186–193.
2. Shaw, J. L., Gislason, G. J., and Imbriglia, J. E. (1958): Transition of cystitis glandularis to primary adenocarcinoma of the bladder. *J. Urol.*, 79:815–822.
3. Koss, L. G. (1979): Mapping of the urinary bladder: its impact on the concepts of bladder cancer. *Hum. Pathol.*, 10:533–548.
4. Ormiston, M. C., Knowles, M. A., Ogbolu, H., Newman, J., Hicks, R. M., and Milroy, E. J. C. (1982): Urothelial abnormalities in the obstructed bladder. *Br. J. Urol.*, 54:234–238.

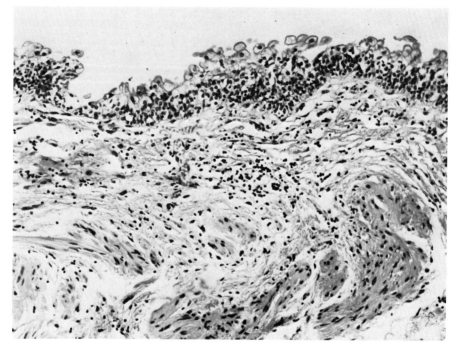

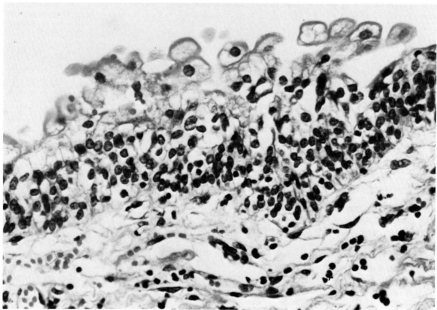

FIGS. 1.1, 1.2. Normal urothelium. ($\times$100 and $\times$200)

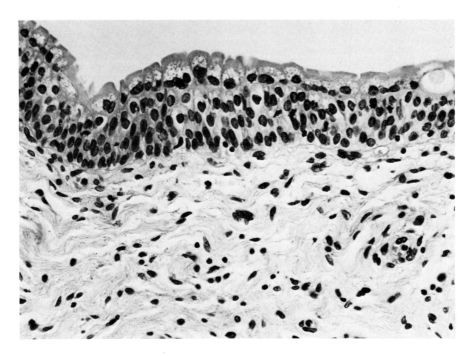

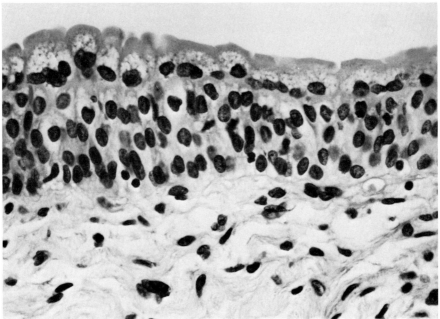

FIGS. 1.3, 1.4. Normal urothelium. (×100 and ×200)

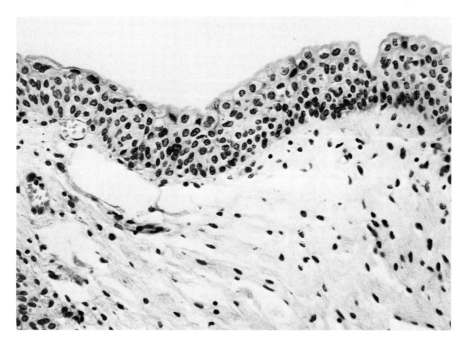

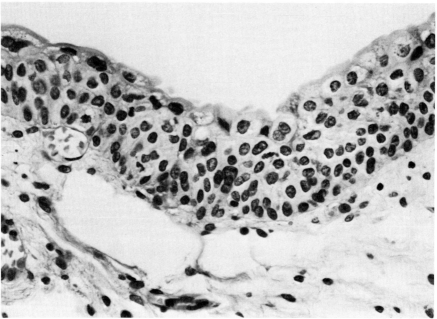

FIGS. 1.5, 1.6. Normal urothelium. ($\times$100 and $\times$200)

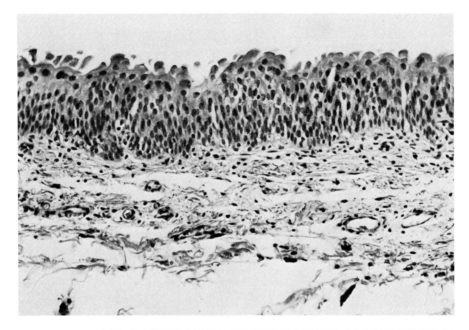

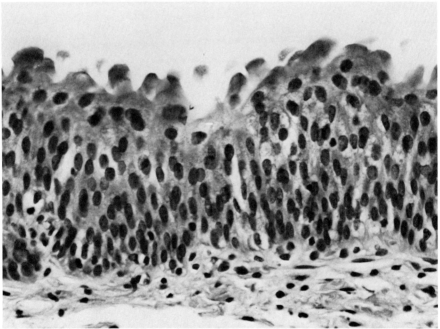

FIGS. 1.7, 1.8. Normal urothelium. ($\times$100 and $\times$200)

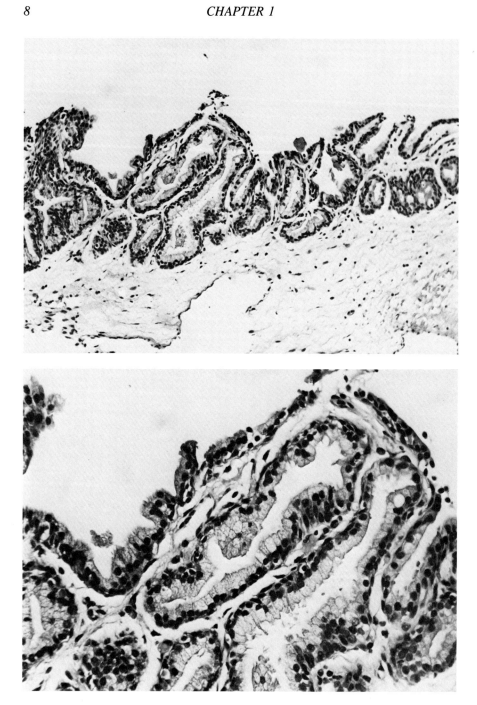

FIGS. 1.9, 1.10.   Normal urothelium of bladder neck. ($\times$100 and $\times$200)

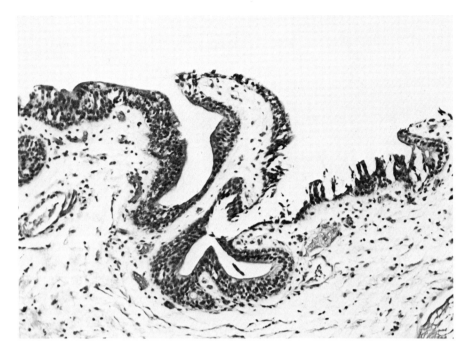

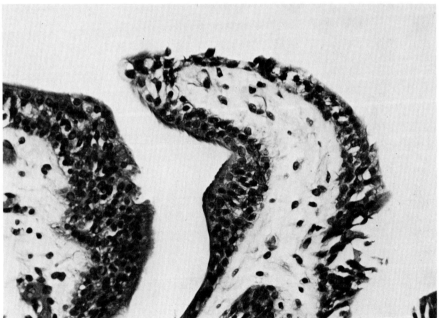

FIGS. 1.11, 1.12. Normal urothelium of bladder neck. (×100 and ×200)

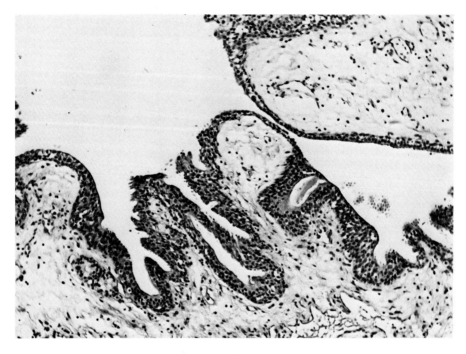

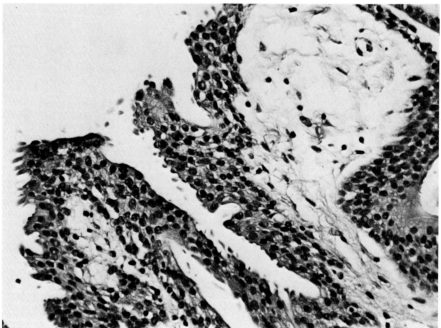

FIGS. 1.13, 1.14. Normal urothelium of bladder neck. ($\times$100 and $\times$200)

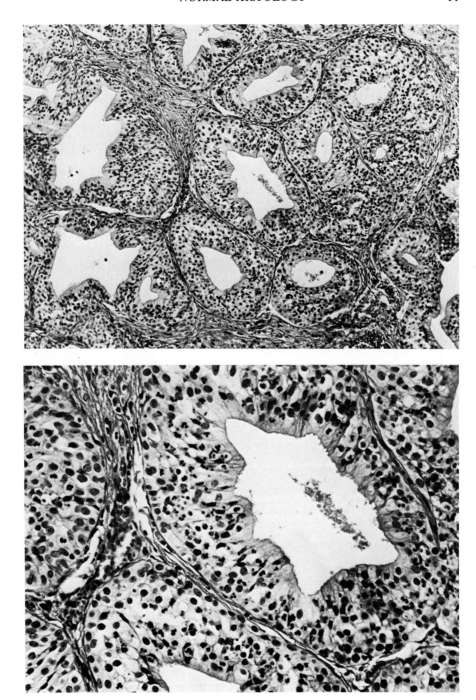

FIGS. 1.15, 1.16. Periurethral ducts of bladder neck. ($\times$100 and $\times$200)

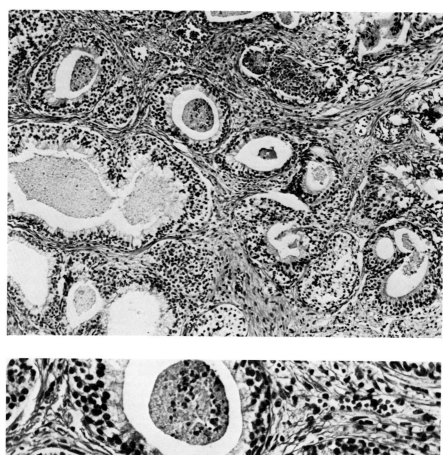

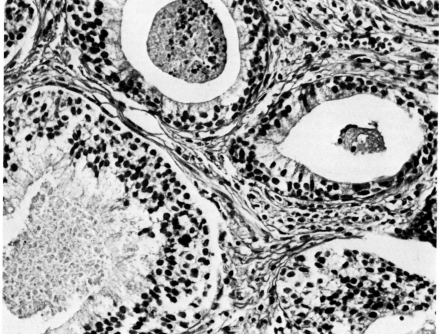

FIGS. 1.17, 1.18. Periurethral ducts of bladder neck. (×100 and ×200)

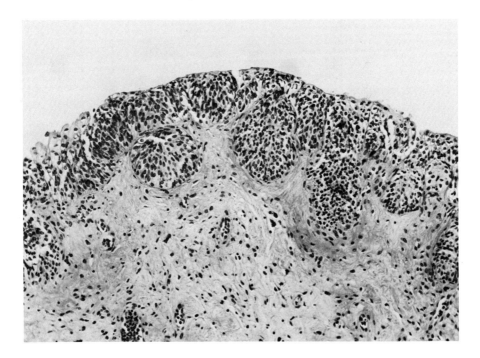

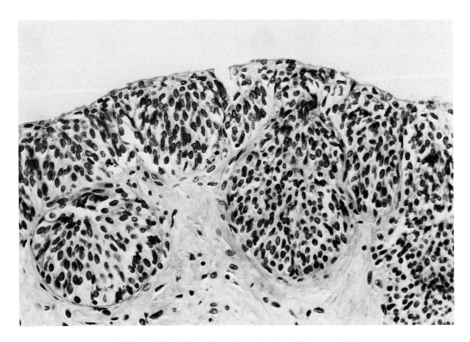

FIGS. 1.19, 1.20.   Brunn's nests. (×100 and ×200)

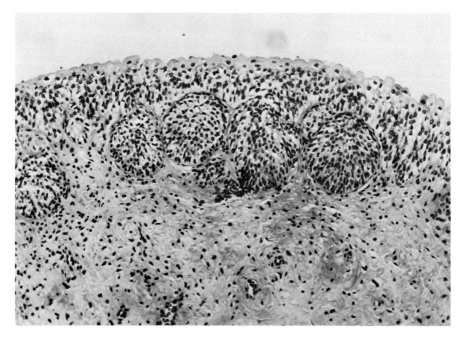

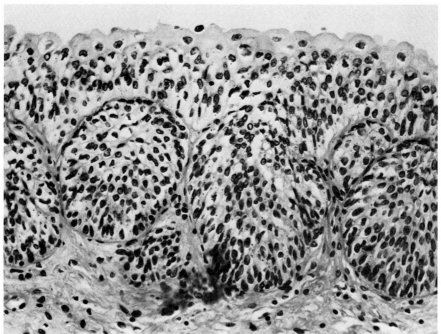

FIGS. 1.21, 1.22. Brunn's nests. (×100 and ×200)

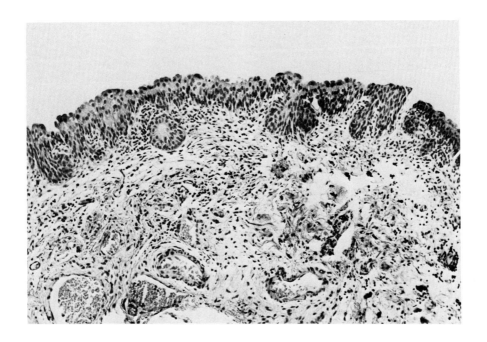

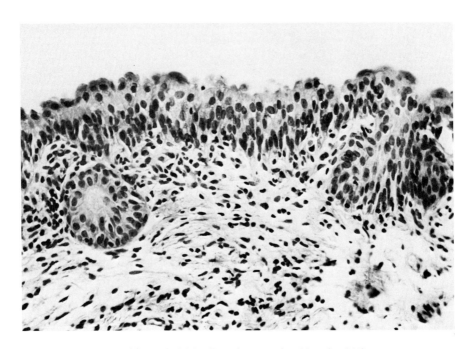

FIGS. 1.23, 1.24. Brunn's nests. (×100 and ×200)

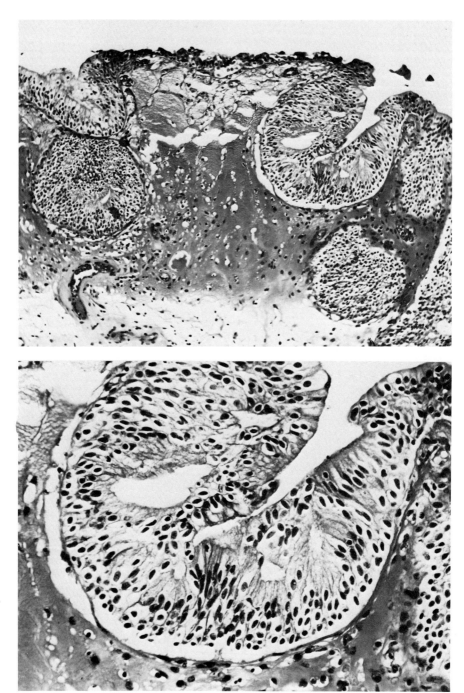

FIGS. 1.25, 1.26. Cystitis glandularis. (× 100 and × 200)

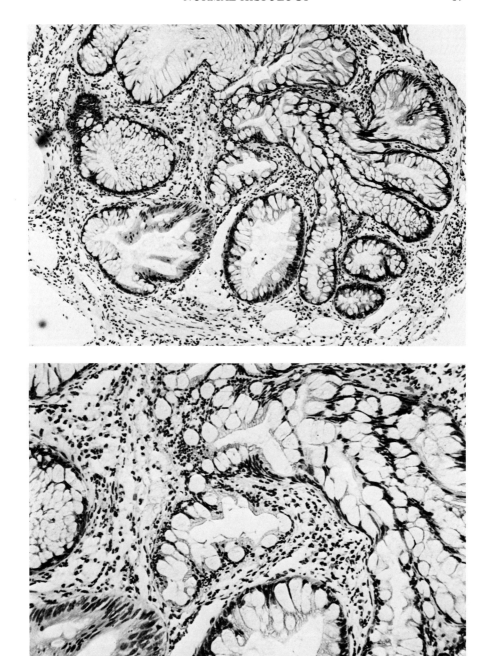

FIGS. 1.27, 1.28. Cystitis glandularis.($\times$100 and $\times$200)

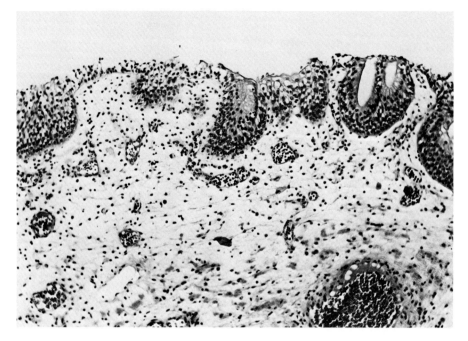

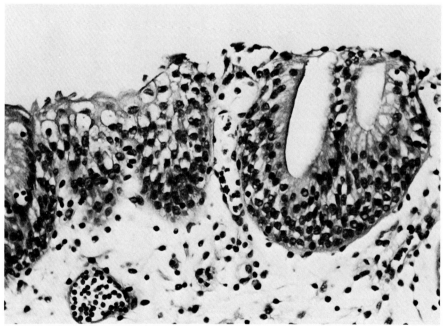

FIGS. 1.29, 1.30. Cystitis cystica. ($\times$100 and $\times$200)

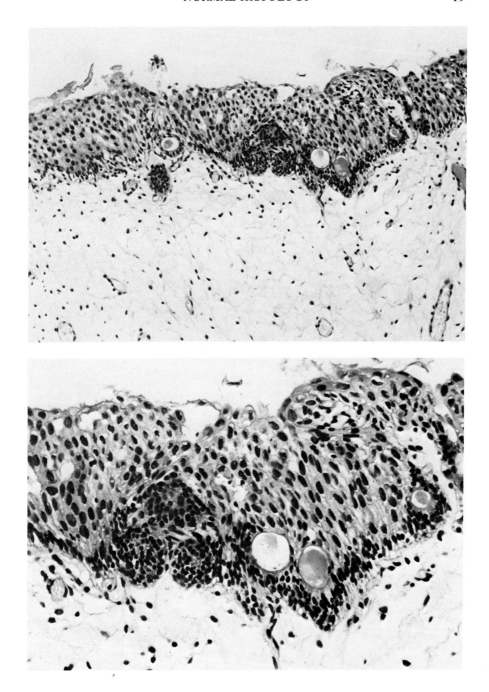

FIGS. 1.31, 1.32. Cystitis cystica. ($\times$100 and $\times$200)

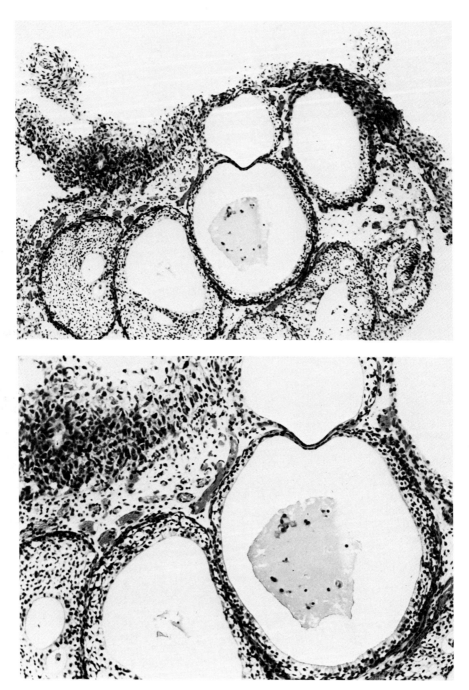

FIGS. 1.33, 1.34.   Cystitis cystica. ($\times 100$ and $\times 200$)

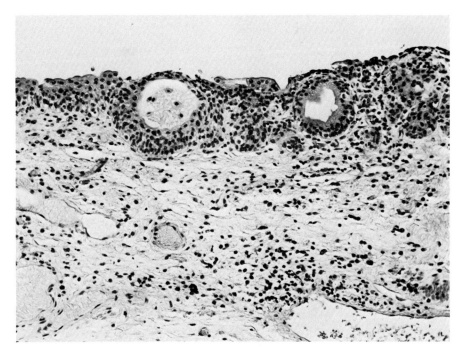

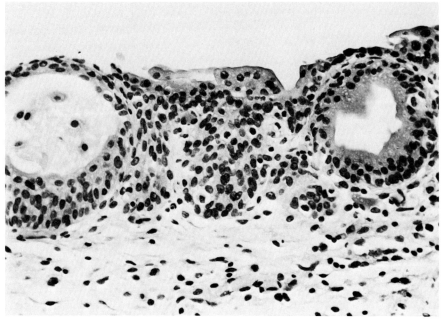

FIGS. 1.35, 1.36. Cystitis cystica. (× 100 and × 200)

Chapter 2

Developmental Abnormalities

EXSTROPHY

Exstrophy is manifested by the absence of the anterior bladder wall and the lower abdominal wall with eversion of the posterior bladder wall. The various forms of this congenital defect are classified according to the degree of malformation. There are two main groups: incomplete and complete. The incomplete, or partial, type is relatively rare and is characterized by the following changes: (a) a defect in the bladder in its lower or upper portion, (b) a relatively slight defect in the abdominal wall, (c) union of the pelvic bones, and (d) normal genitalia. The complete type of exstrophy is more frequently encountered and is characterized by the following: (a) the posterior wall of the bladder protrudes as a reddened, extremely tender mass above the symphysis pubis, (b) lack of development of the lower portion of the anterior abdominal wall, (c) exposed ureteral orifices that constantly bathe the exposed surfaces with urine, (d) separation of the pubic bones, and (e) epispadias in males and cleft clitoris with widely separated labia in females. Other abnormalities such as a rudimentary and stumpy penis, bifid scrotum, undescended testes, bilateral inquinal hernias, and abnormalities affecting the skeleton and gastrointestinal tract often occur.

Exstrophy occurs in approximately every 30,000 to 50,000 births. Over 100 cases are estimated to occur annually in the United States. Males are affected more often than females in a ratio of 2:1 to 7:1. There is no evidence of a familial tendency, although cases have been reported in siblings and identical twins.

Histology

The exposed vesical mucosa, subjected to external contamination and trauma, rapidly undergoes secondary changes. Areas of acute and chronic inflammation, often with areas of acute ulceration and chronic granulation tissue, are almost invariably present. The second most common finding is squamous metaplasia (Figs. 2.1, 2.2), which appears at an early age and becomes more extensive with age. This change, which occurs in approximately 80% of cases, may be so complete as to resemble skin. Proliferative lesions such as cystitis glandularis, cystitis cystica, and Brunn's nests (Figs. 2.3 to 2.6) are found in the majority of cases. It is not always clear whether the glandular elements in exstrophied bladder represent metaplasia or an intrusion of the hindgut into the bladder.

The underlying muscle demonstrates marked fibrosis in 30 to 40% of cases. The fibrosis is encountered more commonly in older patients and seems to be directly dependent on the degree of inflammation. Disorganization in the arrangement of the muscle fibers occasionally occurs.

Course

The upper urinary tracts are normal in the neonate. With time, obstructive changes occur in children with uncorrected bladder exstrophy. The obstruction is almost always caused by fibrosis and metaplasia of the mucosa.

The prognosis of untreated cases is poor because of upper urinary tract infection. Multiple surgical procedures have been utilized to correct the defects of exstrophy. The surgical techniques vary depending on the extent of the exstrophy. Survival to adulthood is not uncommon.

Patients who survive to adulthood are at an increased risk of developing malignant change. Goyanna et al. (1) found 29 cases of carcinoma in exstrophied bladders reported in the literature (Figs. 2.7 to 2.10). Twenty-four of these were adenocarcinomas, two were squamous carcinomas, and three were unidentified carcinomas. Abeshouse (2) reviewed 27 cases of carcinoma developing in exstrophied bladders and found 21 cases of adenocarcinoma, three cases of squamous carcinoma, and three cases of unspecified carcinoma. The patients in Abeshouse's study ranged in age from 23 to 66 with a majority of the carcinomas developing before the age of 50. The carcinomas had a tendency to develop near the apex or superior portion of the protruding bladder mass.

CLOACAL EXSTROPHY (VESICOINTESTINAL FISSURE)

Cloacal exstrophy (Figs. 2.11, 2.12) is a rare anomaly that involves not only the genitourinary system but also the intestinal tract. The characteristic anatomic features are the presence of two hemibladders, each with its own ureter separated by an area of intestine. The incidence is estimated to be 1 in 200,000 live births. Numerous other congenital abnormalities are usually present.

URACHUS

The urachus (Figs. 2.13 to 2.18) is formed from the apical portion of the bladder that reaches the umbilicus in the embryo. As the embryo enlarges, the bladder descends into the pelvic proper, and its apical portion narrows progressively into a fibromuscular strand, the urachus. In adults this fibromuscular strand located between the bladder apex and the umbilicus occasionally retains a central epithelial canal with frequent cystlike dilatations.

Several urachal abnormalities may occur. Among them are:

1. Congenital patent urachus. The urachus remains patent or the apex of the bladder fails to narrow into a fibromuscular duct. Urine exits through both the urethra and umbilicus in this condition.

2. Vesicourachal diverticulum. The urachus is patent only at its vesical termination. The urachus forms a diverticulum opening into the bladder.

3. Umbilical cyst or sinus. The urachal canal opens into the region of the umbilicus. No opening into the bladder is present.

In an autopsy study of 122 adult bladders, residual urachal elements were found in 39 bladders (3). The urachal remnants were observed in the midline on the vertex in 21 cases, on the posterior wall in 17, and on the anterior wall in one. Urachal cysts resulting from focal persistence of the urachus may become infected and present as suprapubic masses. These cysts may depress the dome of the bladder or may rupture and produce peritonitis. The cysts usually present as an intra-abdominal mass filled with an exudate from the epithelial cells.

Histology

The urachus is usually a tubular structure lined by transitional or cuboidal cells. Areas of glandular metaplasia may occur, which result in an epithelium that resembles intestine. The cysts may be dilated or almost occluded. Surrounding the epithelium is a concentric layer of smooth muscle. The smooth muscle is of variable thickness depending on the degree of dilatation of the urachus.

Course

Urachal remnants usually are asymptomatic. Occasionally, they may become dilated with inspissated material causing an abdominal mass. Approximately one-half of all adenocarcinomas primary to the bladder arise from the urachus. Adenocarcinomas of urachal origin tend to occur at an earlier age than adenocarcinomas arising from other areas of the bladder. Some studies (4) have reported a favorable prognosis for urachal adenocarcinomas whereas other studies have shown an extremely poor prognosis (5).

DIVERTICULUM

In children diverticula are almost always congenital. In adults diverticula are usually acquired and are present in 5 to 10% of routine autopsies performed on patients over the age of 50. Diverticula in adults are usually associated with some form of distal obstruction and are found most commonly above the trigone on the posterior wall, the region of the urethral orifice, and the site of the obliterated urachus.

Histology

The urothelium in diverticulum is usually thinner and contains more inflammation than urothelium found elsewhere. Furthermore, in a study at the Mayo Clinic (6), 84% of diverticulum showed dysplastic urothelial changes that at times could be considered frankly premalignant.

Congenital diverticulum retains some musculature in the wall, although it may be thinner than normal. Acquired diverticula have markedly thin musculature or no musculature at all. However, spontaneous perforation of bladder diverticula is extremely uncommon (7).

Course

Diverticula not only have a higher incidence of developing tumors, but the prognosis of tumors developing in diverticula appear to be worse than that of the usual bladder tumor. The Mayo Clinic identified 285 cases of bladder diverticula between 1955 and 1964 (6). In 19 cases (6.7%), a neoplasm had arisen in the diverticulum. The neoplasms all occurred in men, ranging in age from 44 to 84 years, with an average age of 64.3 years. Gross painless hematuria was the initial and only complaint in 15 of the 19 (79%) cases.

Nearly all of the neoplasms developing in the Mayo Clinic study were of the nonpapillary infiltrating type. There were 12 transitional cell carcinomas, six squamous carcinomas, and one leiomyosarcoma. Thirteen of the 19 patients died within the first year of the onset of symptoms and another three patients died during the second year. The average survival period was 11 months.

Due to the risk of malignancy developing in bladder diverticulum, and because bladder diverticulum usually has dysplastic urothelium that at times could be considered frankly premalignant, the Mayo Clinic study "unhesitatingly recommends prophylactic excision of all true diverticula, irrespective of their size, in all patients less than 70 years old, unless compelling medical contraindications exist" (6).

REDUPLICATION

Reduplication is a rare lesion characterized by two bladders separated from one another, lying side by side. Each bladder receives a ureter from its ipsilateral kidney, and each bladder empties through a separate urethra. Reduplication is usually associated with additional congenital abnormalities. There is commonly duplication of the lower gastrointestinal tract.

HYPOPLASIA OR DWARF BLADDER

Hypoplasia, or dwarf bladder, is an extremely rare lesion characterized by extreme reduction in bladder capacity. Hypoplasia is usually associated with other anomalies that are inconsistent with life. Hypoplasia is often recognized at the autopsy table or clinically in later childhood when the patient presents with symptoms of urinary frequency because of extreme reduction in bladder capacity.

AGENESIS

Agenesis is an extremely rare lesion associated with complete absence of the bladder. The ureters may connect with the intestinal tract, vagina, or uterus. Agenesis is usually associated with other congenital abnormalities.

REFERENCES

1. Goyanna, R., Emmett, J. L., and McDonald, J. R. (1951): Exstrophy of the bladder complicated by adenocarcinoma. *J. Urol.*, 65:391–400.
2. Abeshouse, B. S.: Exstrophy of the bladder complicated by adenocarcinoma of the bladder and renal calculi. *J. Urol.*, 49:259–289.
3. Schubert, G. E., Pavkovic, M. B., and Bethke-Bedurftig, B. A. (1982): Tubular urachal remnants in adult bladders. *J. Urol.*, 127:40–42.

4. Thomas, D. G., Ward, A. M., and Williams, J. L. (1971): A study of 52 cases of adenocarcinoma of the bladder. *Br. J. Urol.*, 43:4–15.
5. Mostofi, F. K., Thomson, R. V., and Dean, A. L. (1955): Mucous adenocarcinoma of the urinary bladder. *Cancer*, 8:741–758.
6. Kelalis, P. P., and McLean, P. (1967): The treatment of diverticulum of the bladder. *J. Urol.*, 98:349–352.
7. Mitchell, R. J., and Hamilton, S. G. (1971): Spontaneous perforation of bladder diverticula. *Br. J. Surg.*, 58:712.

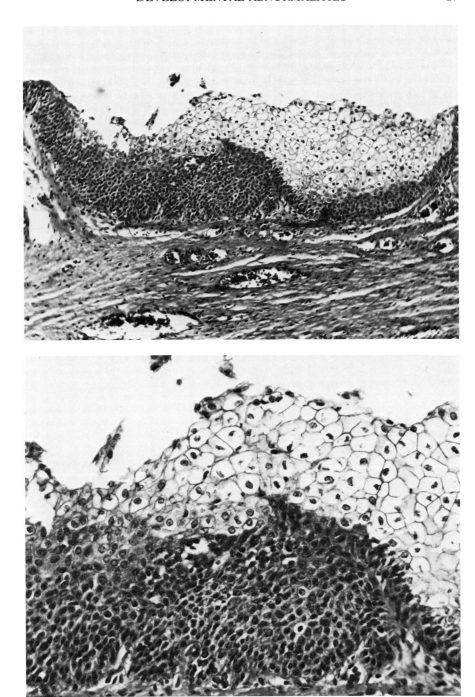

FIGS. 2.1, 2.2. Squamous metaplasia found in exstrophy. ($\times$100 and $\times$200)

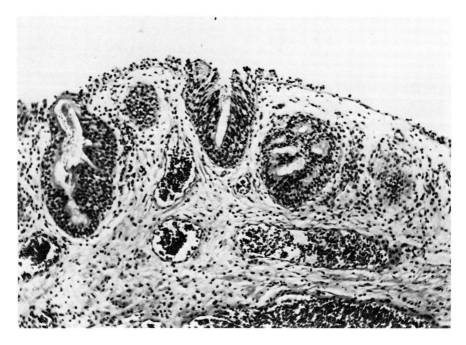

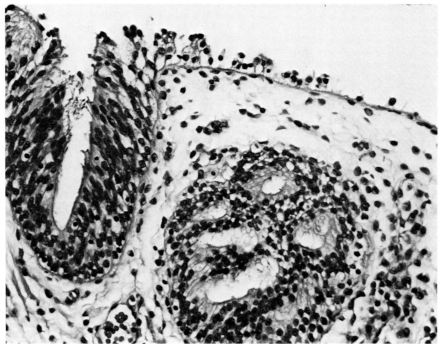

FIGS. 2.3, 2.4. Proliferative lesions found in exstrophy. ($\times$100 and $\times$200)

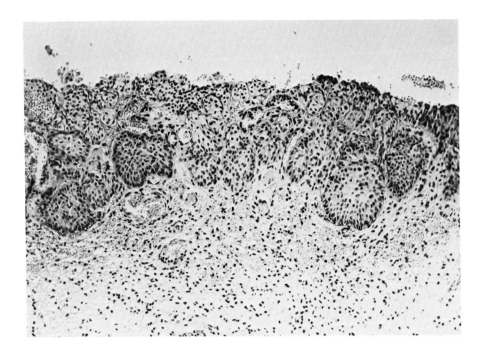

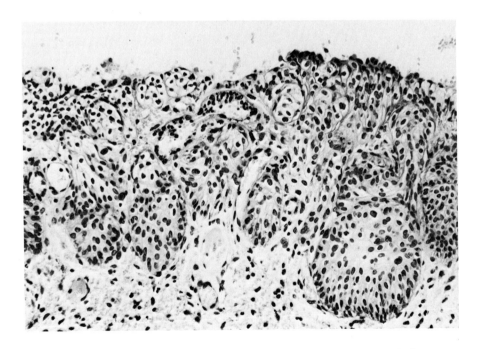

FIGS. 2.5, 2.6. Proliferative lesions found in exstrophy. ($\times$100 and $\times$200)

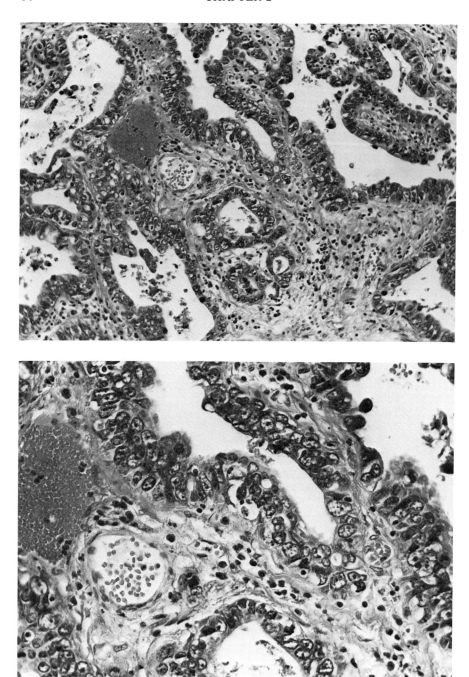

FIGS. 2.7, 2.8.   Adenocarcinoma arising in exstrophy. ($\times$100 and $\times$200)

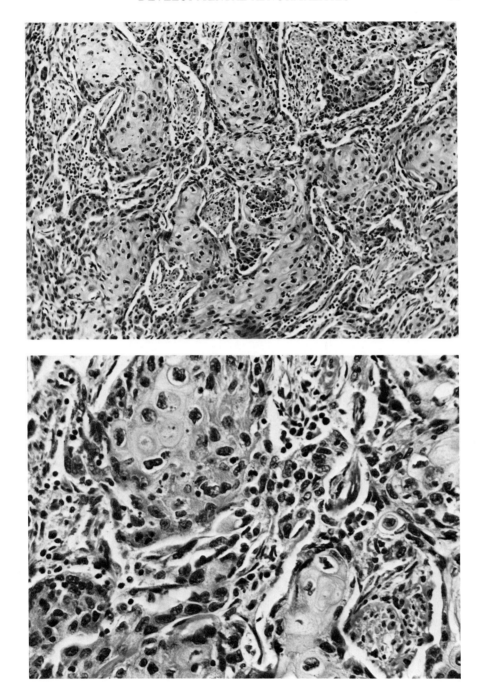

FIGS. 2.9, 2.10. Squamous carcinoma arising in exstrophy. ($\times$100 and $\times$200)

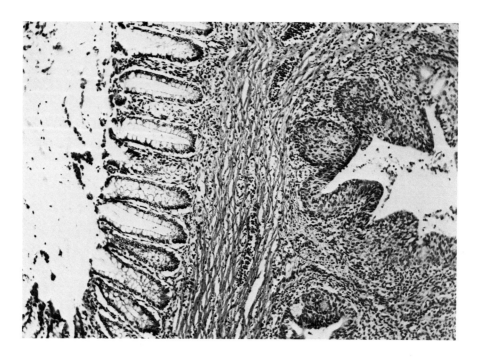

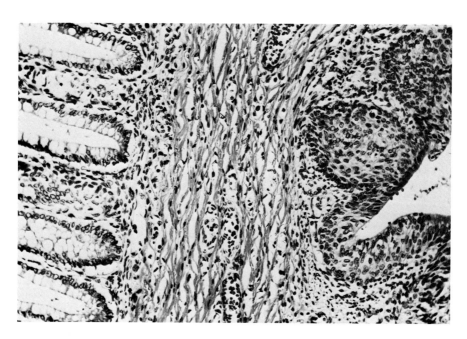

FIGS. 2.11, 2.12. Cloacal exstrophy with colonic mucosa *(left)* and urothelium *(right)*. (×100 and ×200)

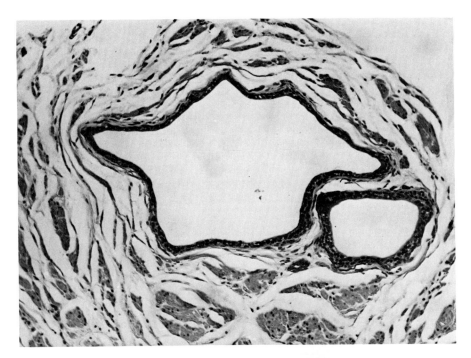

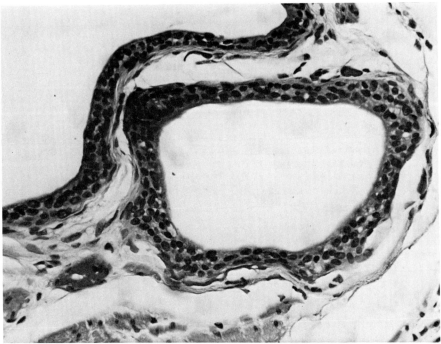

FIGS. 2.13, 2.14. Urachus. (×100 and ×200)

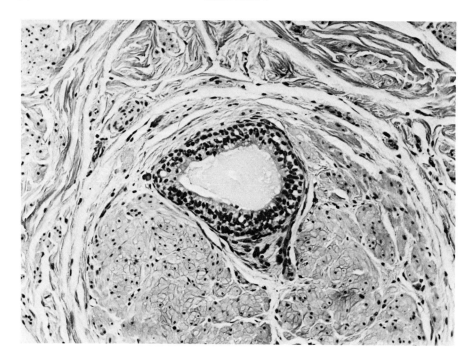

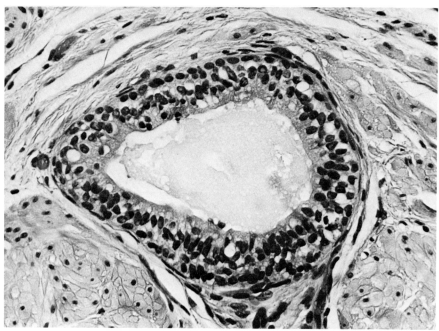

FIGS. 2.15, 2.16.   Urachus. (×100 and ×200)

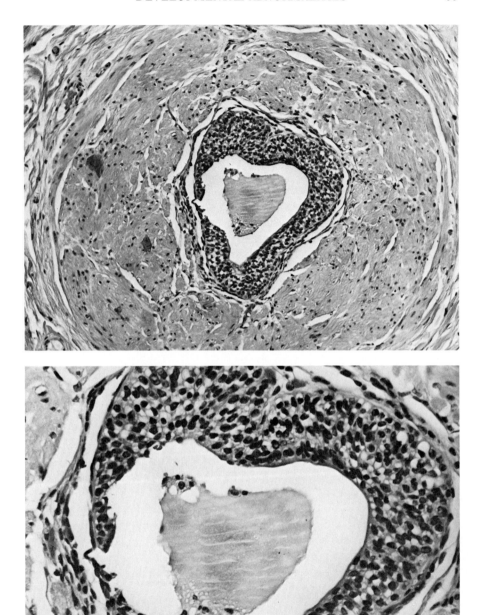

FIGS. 2.17, 2.18 Urachus. ($\times$100 and $\times$200)

Chapter 3

Inflammation

The bladder epithelium is normally resistant to bacterial infection. Cystitis is usually caused by spread of infection from the upper urinary tract, as occurs in tuberculosis, or from the urethra, as occurs when cystitis follows instrumentation. In younger patients, cystitis occurs more commonly in females because of the short urethra that is liable to fecal contamination and to mechanical trauma during intercourse. In older patients, males are affected as frequently as females since prostatic obstruction becomes a frequent cause of cystitis in older males.

ACUTE CYSTITIS

In mild cases of acute cystitis (Figs. 3.1, 3.2), there is mucosal congestion with some local edema and polymorphonuclear leukocyte infiltration. With severe infection, the congestion and edema are pronounced, and the epithelium is either hyperplastic or ulcerated. There is an extensive inflammatory infiltrate composed primarily of polymorphonuclear leukocytes that affect the lamina propria and, not infrequently, the underlying muscular coat. The vasculature of the affected portion of bladder becomes thick walled and the lining endothelium is often prominent.

CHRONIC NONSPECIFIC CYSTITIS

The epithelium in chronic nonspecific cystitis (Figs. 3.3, 3.4) may be eroded, irregularly hyperplastic, or polypoid. In long-term cases, squamous metaplasia is commonly found. The lamina propria becomes thicker with more fibrous tissue than normal. The lamina propria is also congested and diffusely or focally infiltrated with an inflammatory infiltrate that is primarily composed of lymphocytes, plasma cells, and occasional eosinophils and lymphoid follicles. The inflammatory infiltrate commonly extends into the muscular coat. Blood vessels throughout the bladder are usually thickened. The bladder capacity may be reduced in later stages due to contracture caused by proliferation of fibrous tissue.

FOLLICULAR CYSTITIS

Follicular cystitis (Figs. 3.5, 3.6) describes an accumulation of lymphoid follicles in the lamina propria. The mucosa of the bladder, in severe cases, is covered with grayish-red nodules of varying size that may be closely packed together. The nodules are firm on pressure and may be confused with cancer.

Follicular cystitis has been reported more commonly after the age of 50 but may occur at earlier ages. The etiology of these lesions is unknown. Some observers have thought them to be a normal component of the bladder (1). Others have considered them to be a reaction to inflammation, specifically chronic cystitis.

POLYPOID CYSTITIS

"Polypoid cystitis" (Figs. 3.7, 3.8) was a term first used by Friedman and Ash (2) in 1959 to describe a bladder growth that simulated a neoplasm grossly but was considered to be inflammatory, degenerative, and/or reactive in origin. The urothelium may be edematous or hemorrhagic, but more commonly the lesions are only recognized microscopically. Microscopically, the lesions are polypoid, bullous, or papillary with diameters up to 0.5 cm. The underlying lamina propria is usually edematous and congested with a variable amount of inflammatory cells.

These lesions occur with equal frequency in males and females and usually occur after the age of 60. The posterior wall of the bladder is the most commonly affected site. The majority of polypoid cystitis appears to occur in association with indwelling bladder catheters (3). The frequency of this condition increases with prolonged use of the catheter and reaches its peak by 3 months. Polypoid cystitis is what urologists have recognized as "catheter cystitis." Urologists have little difficulty distinguishing polypoid cystitis from tumors, thus explaining why it is rarely biopsied.

EOSINOPHILIC CYSTITIS

Eosinophilic cystitis is characterized by proliferative mucosal lesions that histologically demonstrate an eosinophilic infiltration of the mucosa, submucosa, and/or muscularis. Repeated attacks result in muscle necrosis and fibrosis. The cystoscopic appearance is that of a diffuse edematous and erythematous mucosa with broad based polypoid growths. The mucosal proliferation is not infrequently confused with a bladder tumor at cystoscopy.

Eosinophilic cystitis is characterized by episodes of frequent urination, dysuria, and gross hematuria (4). Eosinophilic cystitis occurs in two different clinical settings. The first is seen in women and children and is often associated with allergic disorders and peripheral eosinophilia. The second presents in older men and is usually associated with bladder injury related to disorders of the bladder or prostate. Parasitic infestation associated with eosinophilic cystitis is rare. This condition is not associated with esosinophilic granuloma (histiocytosis X).

BULLOUS CYSTITIS

Bullous cystitis is a rare form of cystitis in which there is extensive localized edema of the lamina propria and underlying muscularis. This edema results in a folded or polypoid mucosa that appears to form cysts or bullae. These bullae look like grapelike masses directly beneath the mucosal surface. With loss of fluid, these bullae appear as loose, flaccid, wrinkled, low elevations that may grossly resemble the grapelike masses of sarcoma botryoides. The etiology of bullous cystitis is not well understood.

EMPHYSEMATOUS CYSTITIS

Emphysematous cystitis (Figs. 3.9 to 3.12) is a rare condition in which the bladder wall is studded with gas-filled cysts lying in the lamina propria and extending into the superficial muscularis. A foreign-body type of giant cell reaction is characteristically seen at the periphery of the cysts. The gaseous content of the cysts is carbon dioxide.

Emphysematous cystitis develops most often in diabetic patients with glycosuria and/or obstruction or stasis of the urinary tract. Control of the glycosuria has caused a reversal of the lesion. The lesions may also be the result of gas-forming bacteria such as *Escherichia coli* and *Enterobacter aerogenes* within the vesical wall.

HUNNERS ULCER (INTERSTITIAL CYSTITIS)

Hunners ulcers (Figs. 3.13, 3.14) are characterized by submucosal fibrosis with varying numbers of chronic inflammatory cells, including mast cells, and edema. The mucosa is usually ulcerated and covered by fibrin and necrotic material. The lamina propria is thickened, contains increased fibrosis, and is diffusely infiltrated with lymphocytes, plasma cells, polymorphonuclear leukocytes, and eosinophils. The vasculature of the lamina propria is usually dilated or thick-walled. The muscular coat of the bladder has an inflammatory infiltrate, and there may be fibrous replacement of muscle fiber. The lesions occur anywhere in the bladder with no predilection for a specific site. These lesions are one of the least understood entities in bladder pathology. Hunner, in his original description of eight cases in 1915, arrived at a conclusion of nonspecificity for the lesion (5). Hunner's conclusion of nonspecificity has certainly withstood the test of time.

In most series there is a marked predilection for female patients. Most patients are in the 40 to 70 age range. The symptoms are that of lower abdominal, suprapubic, or perineal pain associated with urinary frequency and hematuria (6,7). The symptoms, all unresponsive to medical therapy, may be extremely painful, and they generally progress over several years. Cystoscopy usually shows a hyperemic, contracted bladder that bleeds easily when distended. Pathogenesis has centered around lymphatic obstruction, chronic bladder spasm, and a form of collagen disease.

Males with carcinoma *in situ* of the bladder not infrequently have symptoms similar to those of interstitial cystitis. In a review of 486 patients treated for interstitial cystitis at the Mayo Clinic during a 10-year period, *in situ* cancer of the bladder was identified ultimately in 23% of the men and 1.3% of the women (8). Consequently, males with symptoms of interstitial cystitis should be investigated for the presence of carcinoma *in situ*.

TUBERCULOUS CYSTITIS

The first lesions of tuberculous cystitis (Figs. 3.15 to 3.18) are located about the ureteral orifices. A dense inflammatory infiltrate characterized by granulomas with Langhans giant cells are present. The granulomas initially are small but eventually coalesce and lead to widespread ulceration and contracture of the bladder through extensive fibrosis. The prostate and epididymis are frequently involved.

Most cases (67%) of tuberculous cystitis are the result of seeding of organisms from the upper urinary tract (9). In a study by Wechsler et al. (10), over 50% of the patients developed symptoms before the age of 40. Epididymitis, bladder irritation, and hematuria are the most common symptoms. Most patients have tuberculosis of the kidney, and an even larger percentage have pulmonary tuberculosis.

ACTINOMYCOSIS

Microscopically, actinomycotic granules (Figs. 3.19, 3.20) are found to be up to 25 microns in diameter and surrounded by foamy histiocytes. Polymorphonuclear neutrophils, plasma cells, and fibroblasts form the abscess wall. The center of the granule is basophilic on H&E staining whereas the periphery is composed of tiny, closely packed branching filaments.

Actinomycosis of the bladder is extremely rare. As with tuberculosis of the bladder, actinomycosis on the bladder is usually the result of seeding from the upper urinary tract or from direct extension from adjacent involved viscera. Actinomycosis spreads by burrowing along fascial planes, leaving numerous intercommunications among the sinus tracts.

SCHISTOSOMIASIS

Schistosomiasis (Figs. 3.21 to 3.24) of the bladder is caused by the blood fluke schistosoma hematobium. The blood fluke averages 20 nm in length and 2 nm in width. The eggs are ovoid in shape and are about 50×100 microns. The female blood fluke deposits the eggs in small venules. The eggs develop into larvae that secrete substances that injure the venule. The venule may rupture allowing escape of the embryos into the perivascular tissue of the bladder. The eggs may erode through the bladder mucosa causing perforations and hematuria. The eggs excite an intense inflammatory reaction accompanied by edema and hyperemia.

In some areas of the world, especially Northern Africa, almost the entire population is infected with schistosomiasis. The disease is usually acquired in childhood and is more prevalent in male hosts. Epidemiologically, there appears to be a striking correlation between the incidence of schistosomiasis of the bladder and carcinoma of the bladder. The onset of bladder carcinoma associated with schistosomiasis is at a much younger age in the endemic areas. Dimmette et al. (11) studied 90 cases of carcinoma arising in bladders infested with schistosoma hematobium and found 50 squamous carcinomas, 33 transitional carcinomas, six adenocarcinomas, and one mixed carcinoma (transitional cell carcinoma and adenocarcinoma).

IRRADIATION CYSTITIS

In irradiation cystitis (Figs. 3.25 to 3.30), the bladder may be damaged by local or external radiation applied to the bladder wall or to adjacent organs such as the uterus. The first changes are mucosal congestion and a variable amount of local edema, sometimes progressing to bullae formation. More prolonged exposure produces mucosal ulceration and edema of the lamina propria with acute necrotizing arteriolitis and an inflammatory infiltrate. Vascular thromboses may lead to perforation of the bladder and formation of fistula tracts with the vagina, rectum, or overlying skin. Eventually, fibrosis of the lamina propria and muscle coat leads to contracture of the bladder. Cells exposed to radiation may be enlarged, irregular, and hyperchromatic.

REPARATIVE CYSTITIS

Following injury to the bladder, a reparative process, known as reparative cystitis, develops (Figs. 3.31 to 3.34). Surgery is the most common injury causing the reparative process. The reparative process is characterized by inflammation and fibroblastic proliferation. The fibroblastic proliferation usually takes the form of multinucleated cells that may have cytologically atypical features. These atypical cells may be confused with either new or residual tumor depending on the clinical setting. Consequently, it is important to keep in mind the possible histological changes that can occur in recently injured tissue.

MALAKOPLAKIA

Malakoplakia (Figs. 3.35 to 3.40) is a rare condition that was first described in the urinary tract but has subsequently been found in the testis, epididymis, prostate, and occasionally in the intestine. In the bladder, yellowish, round-to-oval, plague-like or polypoid lesions are scattered over the mucosal surface. Microscopically, the lesions consist of dense collections of large histiocytes with granular cytoplasm called "von Hansemann cells." The von Hansemann cells contain small, rounded, occasionally laminated bodies termed "Michaelis-Gutman bodies" in the cytoplasm or occasionally between the cells. These bodies stain for iron, and with von Kossa and periodic acid-Schiff stains. The Michaelis-Gutman bodies are believed to be altered bacteria or breakdown products of bacteria that have become mineralized (12). Admixed with the histiocytic proliferation is an inflammatory infiltrate composed of polymorphonuclear leukocytes and plasma cells.

FISTULAS

Two types of bladder fistulas between the bladder and female sex organs occur. The most common is a vesicovaginal fistula in which a communication between the bladder and vagina develops. This fistula may occur after obstetric injuries, irradiation damage, severe cystitis, or from direct extension of tumor from one organ to the other. Less commonly, a vesicouterine fistula between the bladder and uterus may develop. Vesicouterine fistulas are caused by similar modalities as vesicovaginal fistulas. The major presenting finding in both fistulas is the escape of urine from the vaginal orifice.

Vesicointestinal fistulas occur between the bladder and the rectum, sigmoid colon, or small bowel. These fistulas are most commonly caused by diverticulitis, tumor, infection, irradiation, or occasionally regional ileitis. Fecal contamination causes passage of turbid urine containing recognizable fecal contents. Urinary obstruction due to fecal material may occur.

Vesicovaginal, vesicouterine, and vesicointestinal fistulas are characterized histologically by inflammatory necrosis of margins of the fistulous tract and severe acute and chronic cystitis.

REFERENCES

1. Alexander, S. (1893): Some observations respecting the pathology and pathological anatomy of nodular cystitis. *J. Cutan. Genitour. Dis.*, 11:245–262.
2. Friedman, N. B., and Ash, J. E. (1959): Tumors of the urinary bladder. AFIP Sect. VI and VIII, Fascicle 31A. Washington, D.C.
3. Ekelund, P., and Johansson, S. (1979): Polypoid cystitis. *Acta Pathol. Microbiol. Scand. (A)*, 87:179–184.
4. Hellstrom, H. R., Davis, B. K., and Shonnard, J. W. (1979): Eosinophilic cystitis. *Am. J. Clin. Pathol.*, 72:777–784.
5. Hunner, G. L. (1914): A rare type of bladder ulcer in women: report of cases. *Trans. Surg. Gynecol. Assoc.*, 27:247–288.
6. Pool, T. L. (1944): Interstitial cystitis: clinical aspects and treatment. *Med. Clin. North Am.*, 28:1008–1015.
7. Smith, B. H., and Dehner, L. P. (1972): Chronic ulcerating interstitial cystitis (Hunners ulcer): a study of 28 cases. *Arch. Pathol.*, 93:76–81.
8. Utz, D. C., and Zincke, H. (1974): The masquerade of bladder cancer in situ as interstitial cystitis. *J. Urol.*, 111:160–161.
9. Auerbach, O. (1940): The pathology of urogenital tuberculosis. *Int. Clin.*, 3:21–61.
10. Wechsler, H., Westfall, M., and Lattimer, J. K. (1960): The earliest signs and symptoms in 127 male patients with genitourinary tuberculosis. *J. Urol.*, 83:801–803.
11. Dimmette, R. M., Sproat, H. F., and Sayegh, E. S. (1956): The classification of carcinoma of the urinary bladder associated with schistosomiasis and metaplasia. *J. Urol.*, 75:680–686.
12. McClurg, F. V., D'Agostino, A. N., Martin, J. H., and Race, G. J. (1973): Ultrastructural demonstration of intracellular bacteria in three cases of malakoplakia of the bladder. *Am. J. Clin. Pathol.*, 60:780–788.

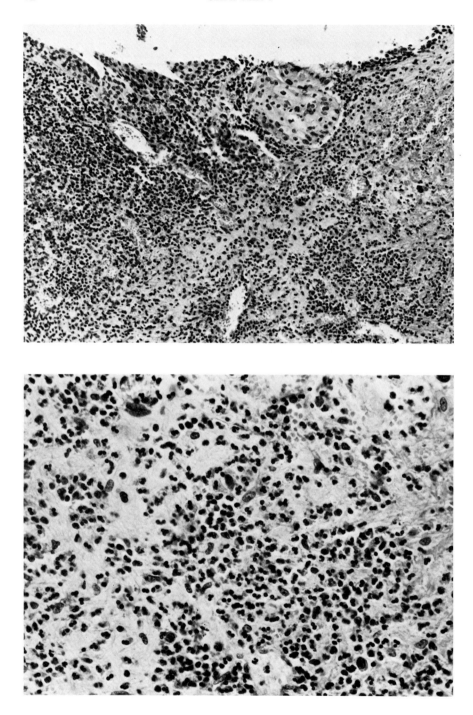

FIGS. 3.1, 3.2. Acute cystitis. ($\times$100 and $\times$200)

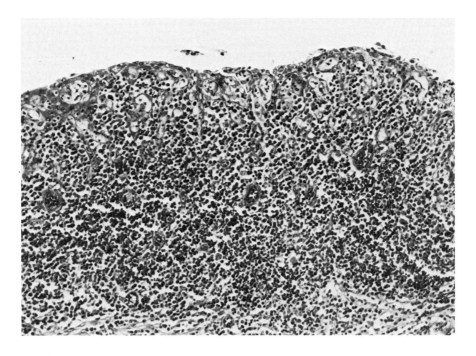

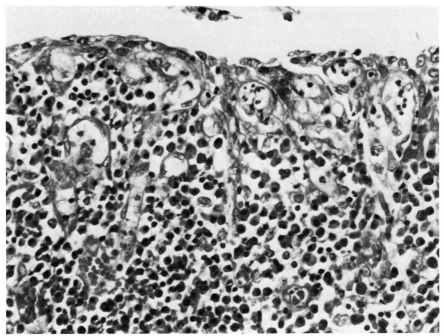

FIGS. 3.3, 3.4. Chronic nonspecific cystitis. ($\times$100 and $\times$200)

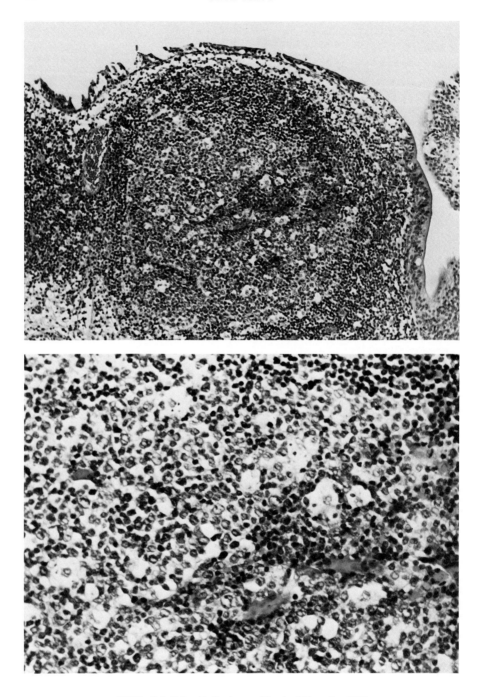

FIGS. 3.5, 3.6. Follicular cystitis. ($\times$100 and $\times$200)

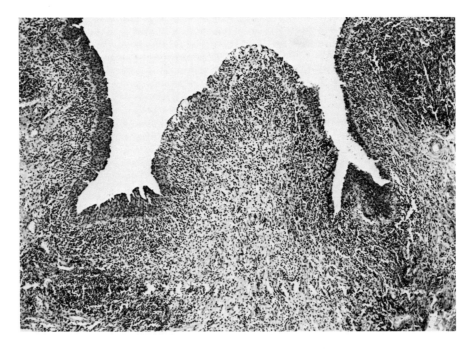

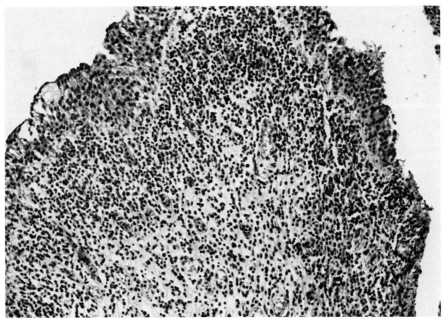

FIGS. 3.7, 3.8. Polypoid cystitis. (×100 and ×200)

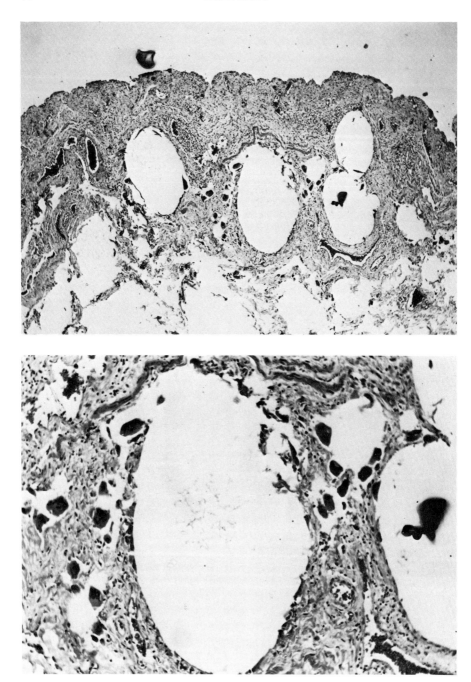

FIGS. 3.9, 3.10   Emphysematous cystitis. ($\times$ 100 and $\times$ 200)

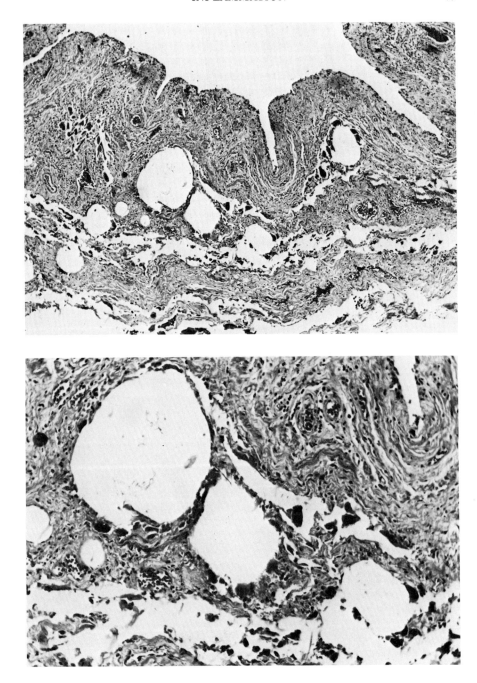

FIGS. 3.11, 3.12. Emphysematous cystitis. ($\times$100 and $\times$200)

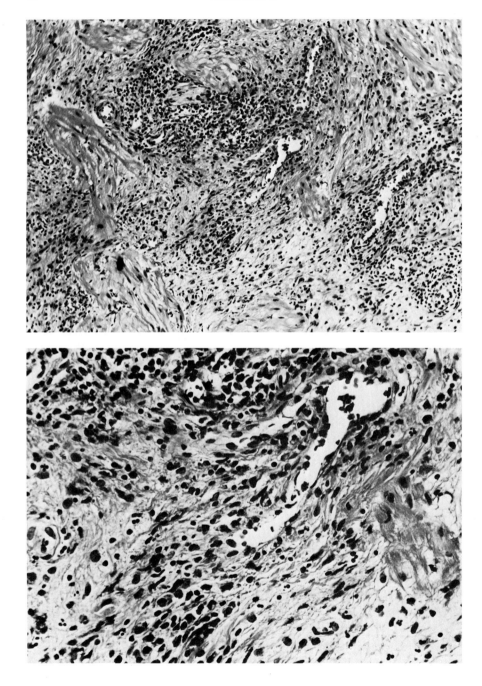

FIGS. 3.13, 3.14.   Hunners ulcer (interstitial cystitis). (× 100 and × 200)

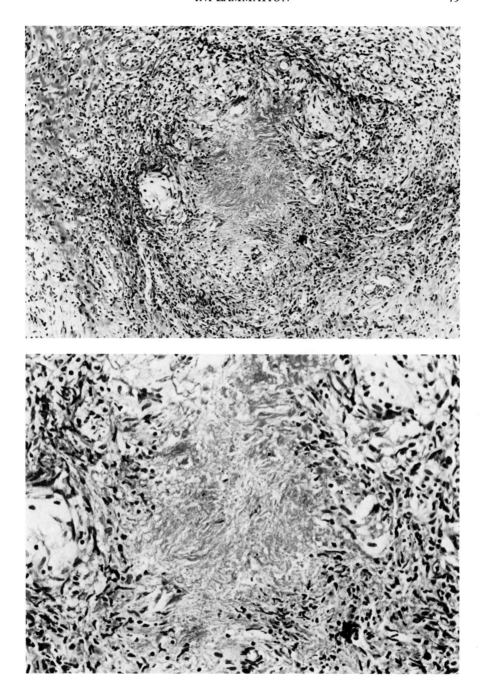

FIGS. 3.15, 3.16. Tuberculous cystitis. ($\times$100 and $\times$200)

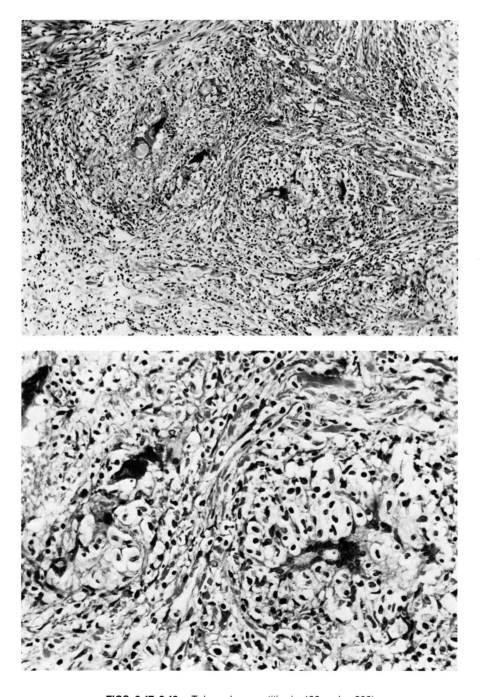

FIGS. 3.17, 3.18. Tuberculous cystitis. ($\times$100 and $\times$200)

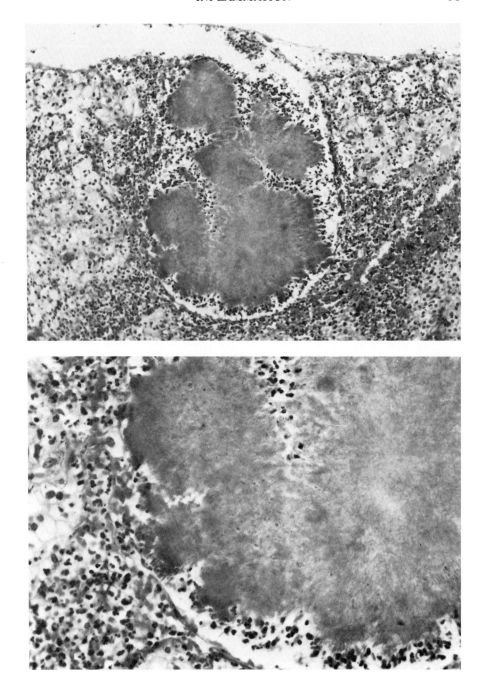

FIGS. 3.19, 3.20. Actinomycosis. ($\times$ 100 and $\times$ 200)

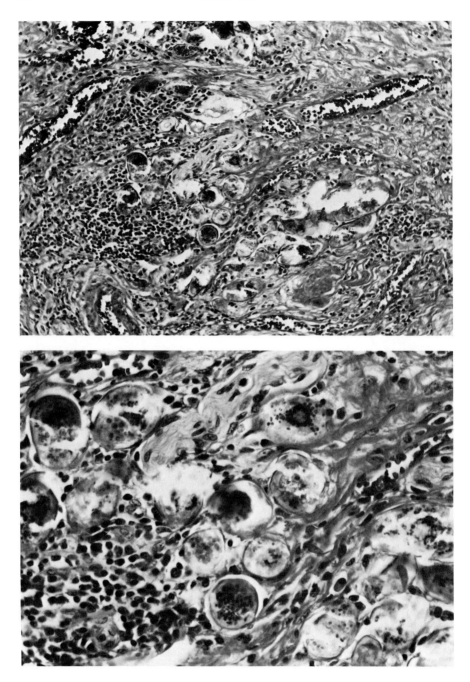

FIGS. 3.21, 3.22. Schistosomiasis. ($\times$ 100 and $\times$ 200)

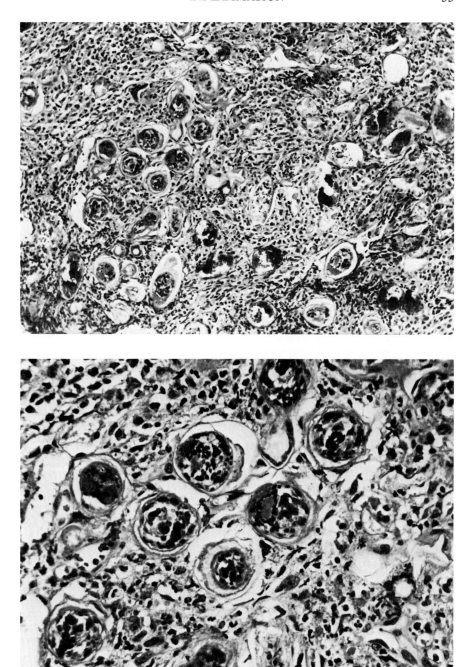

FIGS. 3.23, 3.24. Schistosomiasis. (× 100 and × 200)

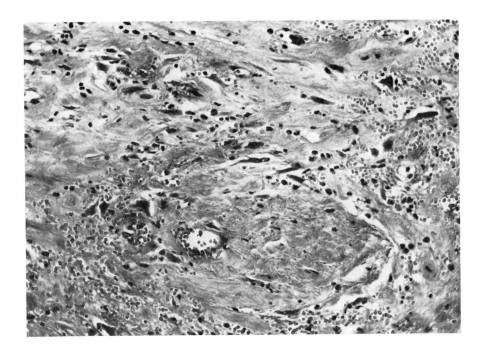

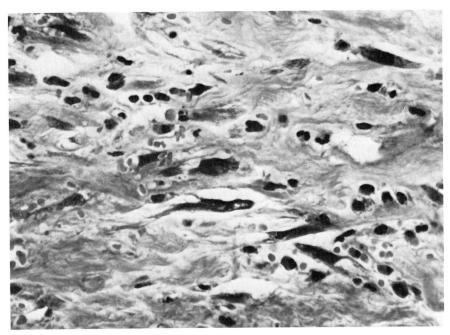

FIGS. 3.25, 3.26.   Irradiation cystitis. ($\times$ 100 and $\times$ 200)

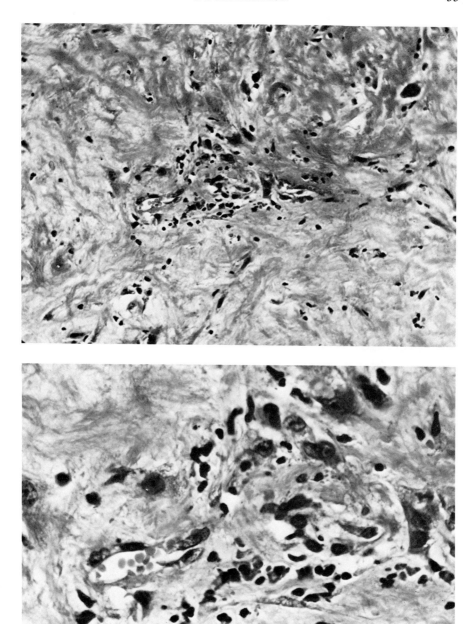

FIGS. 3.27, 3.28. Irradiation cystitis. (× 100 and × 200)

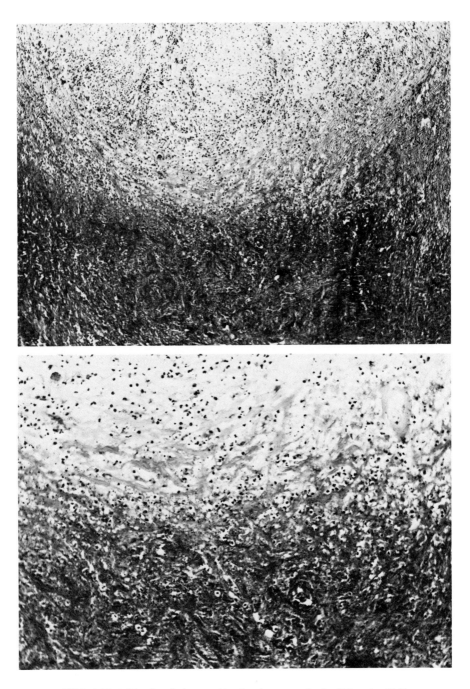

FIGS. 3.29, 3.30. Irradiation cystitis showing necrosis. ($\times$ 100 and $\times$ 200)

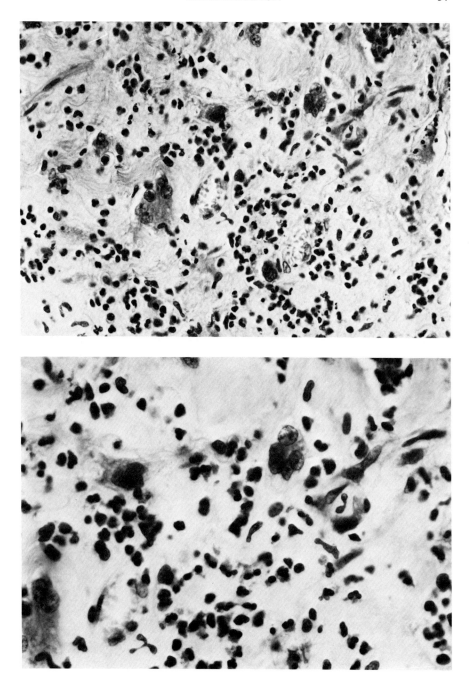

FIGS. 3.31, 3.32. Reparative cystitis. (×200 and ×400)

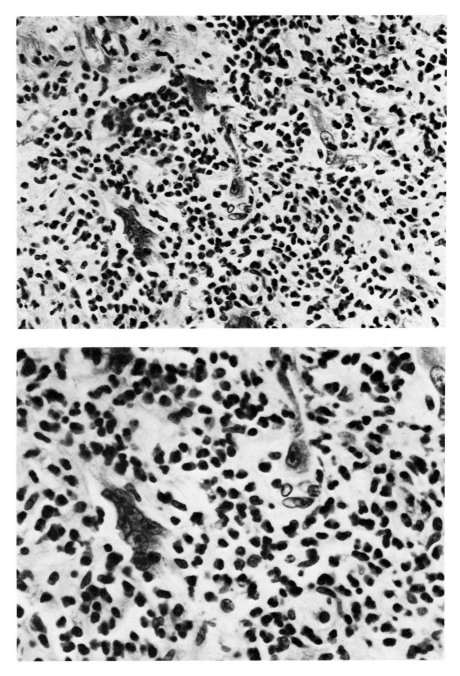

FIGS. 3.33, 3.34. Reparative cystitis. ($\times 200$ and $\times 400$)

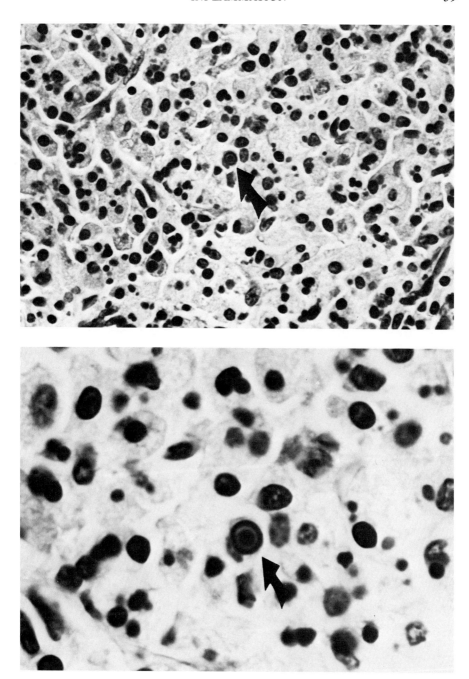

FIGS. 3.35, 3.36. Malakoplakia showing Michaelis-Gutman bodies *(arrow).* (× 400 and × 1000)

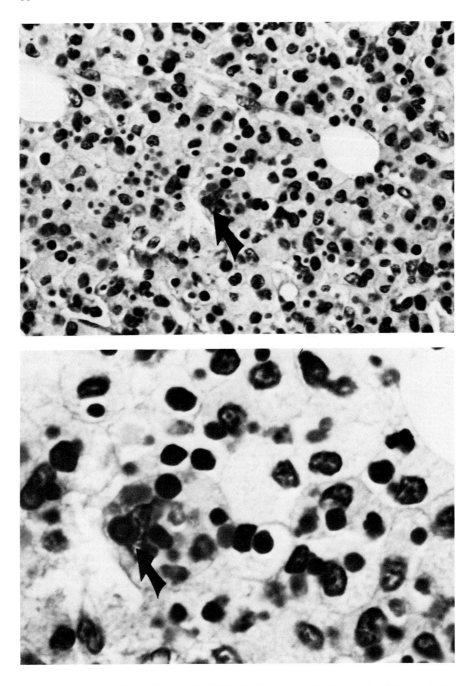

FIGS. 3.37, 3.38. Malakoplakia showing Michaelis-Gutman bodies *(arrow).* ($\times$ 400 and $\times$ 1000)

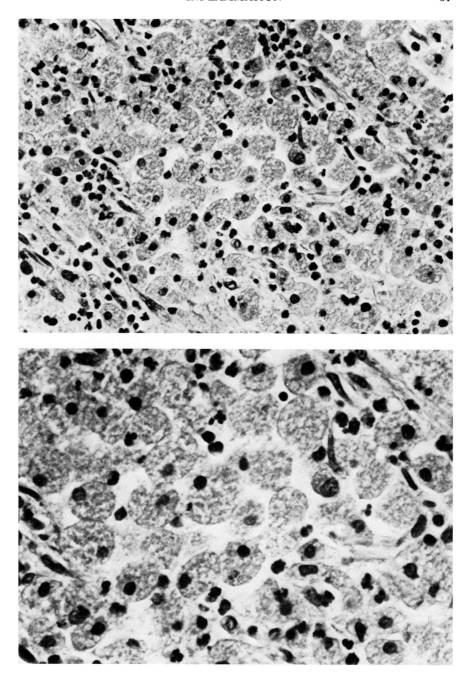

FIGS. 3.39, 3.40. Malakoplakia showing von Hansemann cells. (×200 and ×400)

Chapter 4

Hyperplasia/Dysplasia

Hyperplasias rarely produce recognizable gross lesions in the bladder, and identification of hyperplasia in unselected patient populations has not been feasible. Consequently, it is difficult to study hyperplasia in a pure state by endoscopic localization. To date, most data concerning hyperplasia has been accumulated in patients with known bladder carcinoma. Melicow (1) compared the incidence of hyperplasia in normal and tumor-bearing bladders and found a rare focus of hyperplasia in one of five normal bladders whereas areas of hyperplasia were found in 10 of 10 tumor-bearing bladders. Unfortunately, there have been no large studies that fully document the incidence of hyperplasia in the general population.

SIMPLE HYPERPLASIA

Simple hyperplasia (Figs. 4.1 to 4.6) is characterized by flat urothelium that is increased in thickness. The individual cells show minimal, if any, nuclear abnormalities. The etiologic factors responsible for simple hyperplasia are not clearly understood. There is experimental evidence suggesting that papillary tumors of the bladder begin as areas of hyperplasia. However, in humans, it is not known with certainty whether simple hyperplasia is occasionally a premalignant lesion or a lesion with no oncological significance whatsoever.

PAPILLARY HYPERPLASIA

"Papillary hyperplasia" (Figs. 4.7 to 4.10) is a term that has been used to describe urothelium having a tendency to produce low, broad papillary processes that project into the bladder lumen. Papillary hyperplasia can be distinguished from papillary transitional cell tumors by the presence of broad, regular papillary projections that are only slightly elevated above the surrounding urothelium.

ATYPICAL HYPERPLASIA/DYSPLASIA

Atypical hyperplasia of the bladder (Figs. 4.11 to 4.22) is often termed "dysplasia." Atypical hyperplasia/dysplasia describes histological changes between normal and carcinoma *in situ*. According to the severity of disturbance seen, these lesions are described as mild, moderate, or severe.

Atypical hyperplasia/dysplasia is defined as having some or all of the following characteristics: deviation of nuclear size, shape and staining, loss of orderly cell arrangement with more or less clumping of cells and nuclei, prominent nucleoli, increased mitoses, increased nuclear to cytoplasmic ratio resulting in the appearance of cell crowding, loss of cell polarity, and increase in nuclear hyperchromasia. An increase in the thickness of the urothelium is not always present. The changes are first seen in the basal and intermediate cells, which continue to have a continuous covering of normal-appearing superficial cells. Severe dysplasia approaches the changes seen in carcinoma *in situ*. The major differences between dysplasia and carcinoma *in situ* are a lack of full thickness involvement of the urothelium and a slightly less degree of nuclear pleomorphism and hyperchromasia in dysplasia. These differences are often subjective and the diagnosis in a particular case often depends on the individual judgment of the surgical pathologist.

SIGNIFICANCE OF HYPERPLASIA/DYSPLASIA

Numerous experimental studies indicate that the development of invasive carcinoma of the urinary bladder is usually preceded by hyperplasia and dysplasia of the urothelium. Littlefield et al. (2) found a highly significant correlation between persistant hyperplasia of the urothelium and the subsequent incidence of bladder cancer in animal studies. However, hyperplasia/dysplasia in humans has been more difficult to study in a pure state. Nonetheless, these lesions have attracted considerable attention. Friedman and Ash in 1959 first suggested that hyperplastic lesions may be more than a curiosity by stating "abnormal epithelial patches in the lining near tumors have been described and may be of importance in the genesis of subsequent tumors" (3). L. G. Koss furthered this concept by stating "the nonpapillary epithelial abnormalities, such as atypical hyperplasia and nonpapillary carcinoma *in situ*, are the common source of invasive bladder carcinoma" (4).

There is considerable evidence supporting Koss's viewpoint. Althausen et al. (5) studied 78 patients with noninvasive papillary lesions. Invasive carcinomas developed in 7% of the patients when the surrounding urothelium was normal whereas invasive carcinoma developed in 36% of patients when the surrounding urothelium was atypical.

Eisenberg (6) also demonstrated the prognostic significance of hyperplasia in a study of noninvasive papillary tumors. In Eisenberg's study, patients with noninvasive papillary tumors had no recurrences when the surrounding urothelium was normal. However, all of the cases which died of invasive bladder carcinoma had proliferative lesions, including hyperplasia, in urothelium surrounding the noninvasive papillary tumors.

The studies of Althausen et al. and Eisenberg et al. suggest that the presence of hyperplasia, atypical hyperplasia, or dysplasia adjacent to a noninvasive papillary tumor is an indication that the entire urothelium is likely to be in a state of unrest, which may occasionally manifest itself as invasive bladder carcinoma. Although most dysplastic lesions apparently do not progress, the frequency of the association between dysplastic lesions and subsequent invasive carcinoma is sufficiently high to suggest that dysplasia is a significant risk factor. Consequently it would seem prudent to place these patients in a category of elevated risk, in which they should be followed by cytology and cystoscopic studies at regular intervals.

REFERENCES

1. Melicow, M. M. (1952): Histological study of vesical urothelium intervening between gross neoplasms in total cystectomy. *J. Urol.*, 68:261–279.
2. Littlefield, N. A., Greenman, D. L., and Farmer, J. H. (1979): The effects of continuous and discontinued exposure to 2-AAF on urinary bladder hyperplasia and neoplasia. *J. Environ. Pathol. Toxicol.*, 3:35–54.
3. Friedman, N. B., and Ash, J. E. (1959): Tumors of the urinary bladder. AFIP, Sect. VI and VIII, Fascicle 31A, Washington, D.C.
4. Koss, L. G. (1979): Mapping of the urinary bladder. *Hum. Pathol.*, 10:533–548.
5. Althausen, A. F., Prout, G. R., and Daly, J. J. (1976): Noninvasive papillary carcinoma of the bladder associated with carcinoma in situ. *J. Urol.*, 116:575–580.
6. Eisenberg, R. B., Roth, R. B., and Schweinberg, M. H. (1960): Bladder tumors and associated proliferative mucosal lesions. *J. Urol.*, 84:544–550.

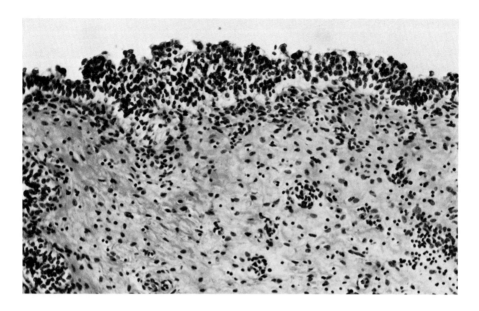

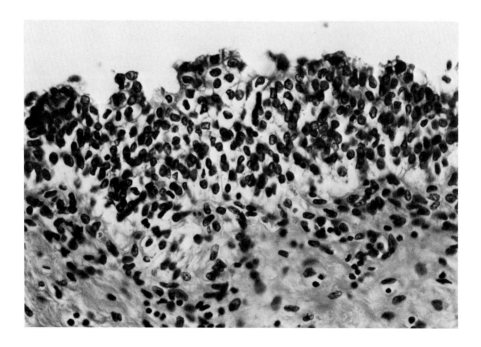

FIGS. 4.1, 4.2. Simple hyperplasia. (×100 and ×200)

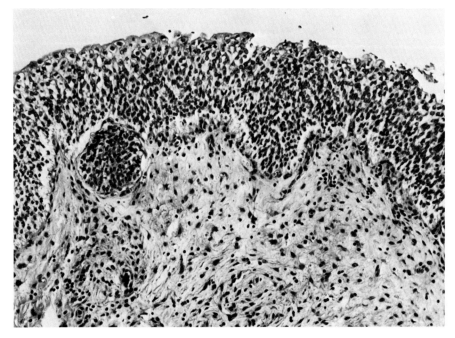

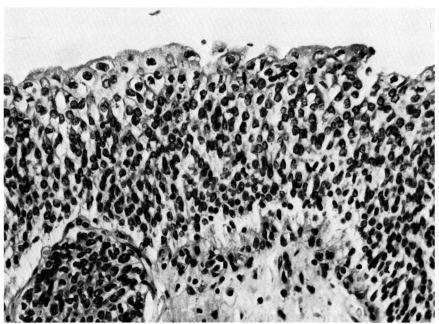

FIGS. 4.3, 4.4. Simple hyperplasia. (×100 and ×200)

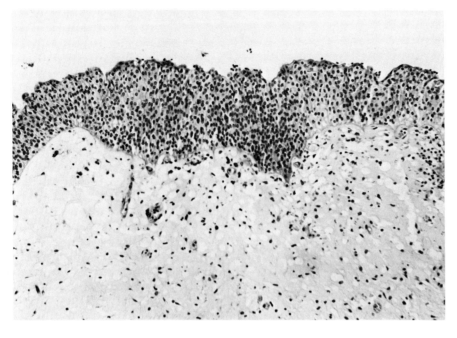

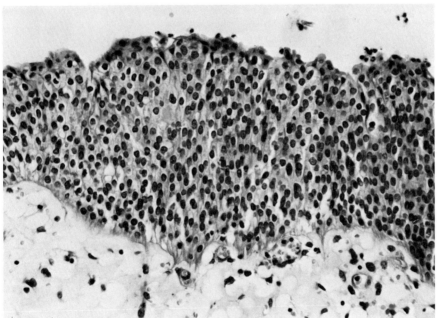

FIGS. 4.5, 4.6. Simple hyperplasia. (×100 and ×200)

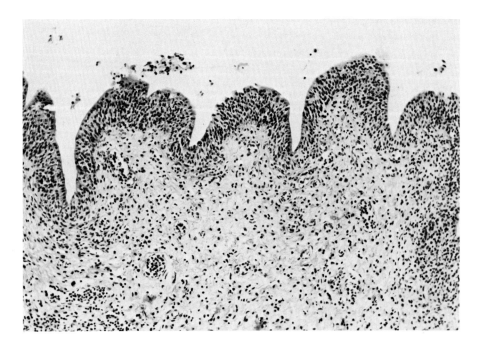

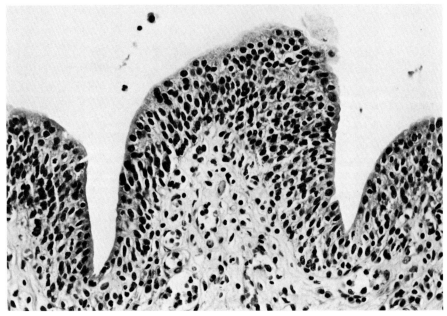

FIGS. 4.7, 4.8. Papillary hyperplasia. ($\times$100 and $\times$200)

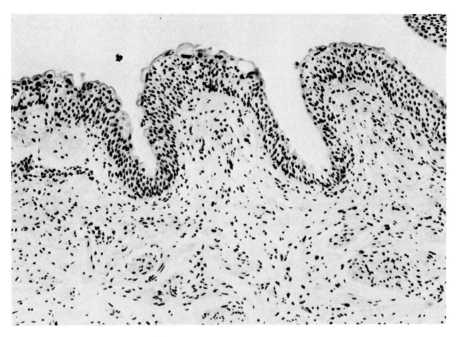

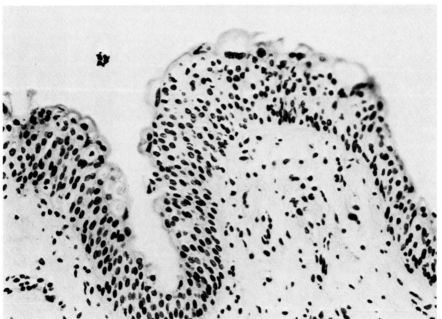

FIGS. 4.9, 4.10. Papillary hyperplasia. (×100 and ×200)

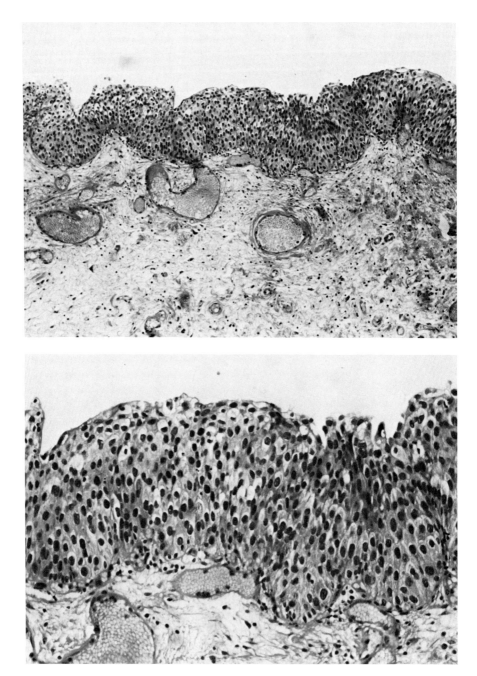

FIGS. 4.11, 4.12.   Atypical hyperplasia. (× 100 and × 200)

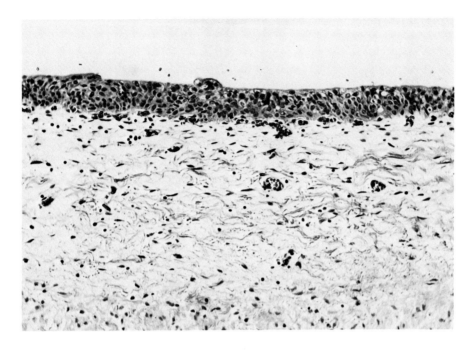

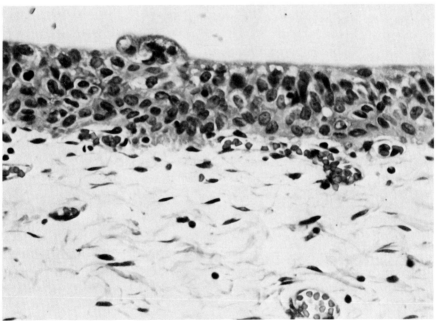

FIGS. 4.13, 4.14. Atypical hyperplasia. (×100 and ×200)

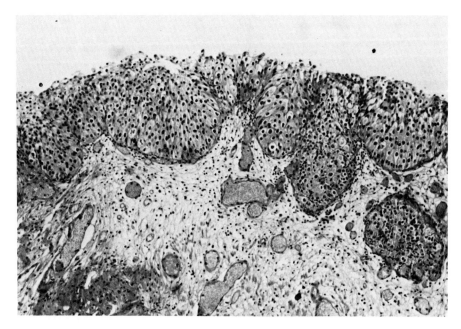

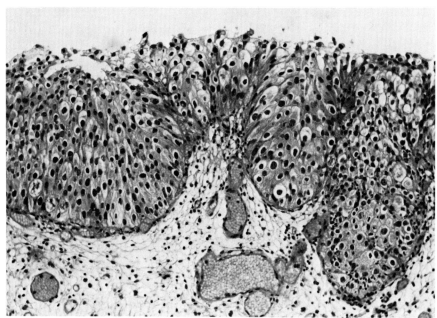

FIGS. 4.15, 4.16. Atypical hyperplasia. ($\times$100 and $\times$200)

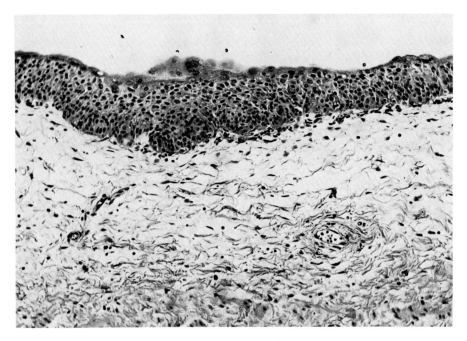

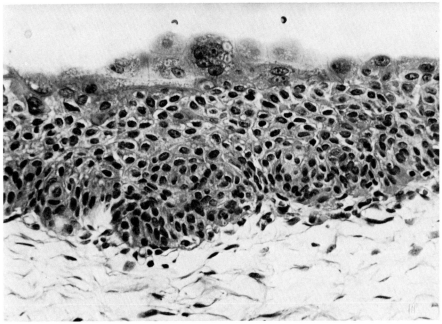

FIGS. 4.17, 4.18. Atypical hyperplasia. ($\times 100$ and $\times 200$)

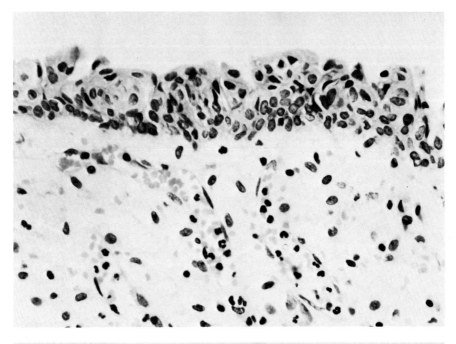

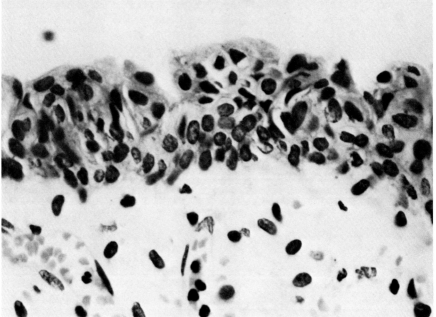

FIGS. 4.19, 4.20. Atypical hyperplasia approaching carcinoma *in situ*. (×100 and ×200)

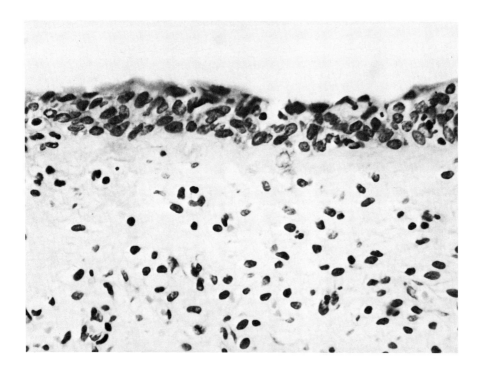

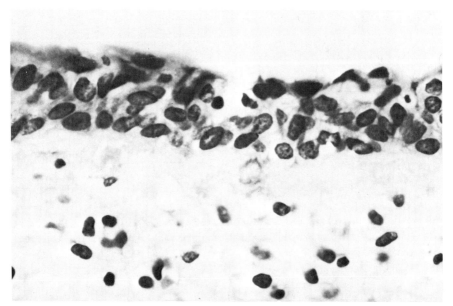

FIGS. 4.21, 4.22. Atypical hyperplasia approaching carcinoma *in situ.* (×100 and ×200)

Chapter 5

Introduction to Bladder Tumors

Bladder tumors are usually divided into three major groups. The most frequent are transitional cell tumors. Second in frequency are squamous carcinomas. Adenocarcinomas are the third and least frequent type.

Transitional cell tumors are divided into papillary and nonpapillary types. Papillary transitional cell tumors are usually divided into four groups. When the lining urothelium shows limited atypia with normal or slightly increased thickness, the lesion is designated a papilloma. Papillary carcinomas are divided into Grades 1, 2, and 3 with the degree of nuclear abnormalities and the likelihood of invasion increasing with increasing grade.

Nonpapillary transitional cell tumors are divided into carcinomas *in situ* and invasive nonpapillary carcinomas. Carcinoma *in situ* may occur as a primary disorder or may occur in urothelium adjacent to a papillary or invasive lesion. Carcinoma *in situ* demonstrates no evidence of invasion, and the malignant alterations are limited to the urothelium. Invasive nonpapillary carcinomas involve the underlying lamina propria and/or muscle wall.

Squamous carcinomas account for 3 to 5% of all bladder carcinomas in the Western world. In Eastern Africa, particularly Egypt, squamous carcinoma is the most common bladder malignancy and is associated with infestation with schistosoma hematobium.

Adenocarcinoma of the bladder is the least common type of carcinoma of the bladder. Adenocarcinomas primary to the bladder may originate in remnants of the urachus, from an exstrophic bladder, or occasionally appear to develop from altered urothelium, such as cystitis glandularis or cystitis cystica.

MODE OF PRESENTATION OF INVASIVE BLADDER CARCINOMA

There has been a widely held idea that the majority of invasive carcinomas of the bladder occur in patients with a history of papillary neoplasms of the bladder. Papillary neoplasms of the bladder are commonly thought to recur over many years with a tendency toward increasing pleomorphism until an invasive bladder carcinoma develops. However, there has been increasing speculation that papillary neoplasms of the bladder are rather innocuous lesions that merely indicate that other nonpapillary areas of the urothelium may be in a malignant or premalignant condition. In fact, L. G. Koss (1) has stated that:

> papillary tumors may have "pushy margins" which extend to the lamina propria and compress the muscularis but rarely invade the muscularis and thus are relatively

innocuous to the patient. The nonpapillary epithelial abnormalities, such as atypical hyperplasia and nonpapillary carcinoma *in situ*, are the common source of invasive bladder carcinoma.

In support of Koss's concepts, several studies have shown that the vast majority of invasive bladder carcinomas occur without a history of papillary neoplasms. Brawn (2) studied 104 consecutive cases of invasive bladder carcinoma and found that 84 (80%) of the cases presented without a history of papillary neoplasms whereas only 20 of the 104 cases had a history of papillary neoplasms. Furthermore, 22 of the 84 cases that did not have a history of papillary lesions had cystoscopies performed months to years prior to the diagnosis of invasive bladder carcinoma. These cystoscopies failed to identify papillary neoplasms of the bladder.

Kaye and Lange (3) analyzed the medical histories of 166 patients with invasive bladder carcinoma and found that only 16% had prior noninvasive bladder tumors. Kaye and Lange concluded that the majority of patients who will ever have invasive bladder carcinoma will already have it when first seen.

Brawn (4) followed 10 patients with noninvasive papillary lesions who subsequently developed invasive bladder carcinoma. All cystoscopy reports and all tissue removed for histological study were available for review. Five of the 10 patients developed an invasive bladder carcinoma in a location distinctly separate from any preceding papillary lesion. The remaining five patients developed an invasive lesion in the same general location as a preceding papillary lesion. Whether these latter five invasive lesions developed directly from the preceding papillary lesion or developed in urothelium adjacent to the papillary lesion could not be determined with certainty. Brawn concluded:

> . . . not only do the vast majority of invasive bladder carcinomas arise without a history of papillary lesions but the occasional invasive bladder carcinoma which develops in a bladder with a history of papillary lesions often develop[s] in a location distinctly separate from any preceding papillary lesion[s].

There is considerable experimental data supporting the concepts of L. G. Koss. Although papillary tumors are readily induced in experimental animals, invasive papillary tumors are uncommon and are seen only after prolonged periods of large doses of carcinogens (5–8). However, experimentally induced invasive bladder carcinomas are much more commonly of the keratinized type and usually develop from "flat" epithelium rather than from papillary lesions (8).

At present, evidence suggests that therapeutic gains in bladder cancer might follow from improved screening methods for asymptomatic patients and wider application of the screening methods. Vigorously attacking the highly visible papillary neoplasm may not be as fruitful in preventing invasive bladder carcinoma as attempting to identify the presence of nonpapillary lesions of the bladder, which appear to be the most frequent precursors of invasive bladder carcinoma.

IDENTIFICATION OF PATIENTS AT RISK OF DEVELOPING INVASIVE BLADDER CARCINOMA

Approximately 10% of patients with noninvasive papillary lesions will eventually develop invasive bladder carcinoma whereas 90% will not (9,10). The subsequent invasive lesions usually develop from atypical changes in the surrounding urothelium rather than directly from the preceding noninvasive papillary lesion that has been completely removed. There are several methods that have been utilized to identify those patients with noninvasive papillary lesions who are at a high risk of developing invasive bladder carcinoma.

Random Biopsies

Eisenberg et al. (11) in 1960 first demonstrated that patients with noninvasive papillary lesions who subsequently develop invasive bladder carcinoma are likely to have histological abnormalities in the urothelium adjacent to the papillary lesion. In Eisenberg's study, those patients with noninvasive papillary lesions who subsequently developed invasive bladder carcinoma all had abnormal urothelium (hyperplasia, dysplasia, carcinoma *in situ*) adjacent to the noninvasive papillary lesion whereas those patients who did not develop invasive carcinoma had normal urothelium surrounding the noninvasive papillary lesion.

Althausen et al. (12), found that only three of 41 (7%) patients with noninvasive papillary lesions subsequently developed invasive bladder carcinoma when the urothelium surrounding the papillary lesion was normal. However, nine of 25 (36%) patients with atypia and 10 of 12 (83%) patients with carcinoma *in situ* in the urothelium surrounding the noninvasive lesions subsequently developed invasive bladder carcinoma.

Wolf and Hojgaard (13) have shown that the histology of the flat urothelium surrounding invasive lesions is of prognostic significance. They followed 25 patients with tumors invading the lamina propria or having invasion of the superficial muscle who fulfilled the following criteria:

1. They were treated primarily only with transurethral resection of the tumor.
2. They had random preselected site mucosal biopsies performed at the initial diagnosis.
3. They had been followed for at least 12 months.

Wolf and Hojgaard found that when urothelial dysplasia was absent in the surrounding urothelium, only two of 17 patients developed new tumors during the period of observation. When urothelial dysplasia was present in the surrounding urothelium, eight of nine patients developed new tumors within the period of observation. They concluded that the presence of urothelial dysplasia concomitant to an infiltrating bladder tumor at the initial diagnosis seems to be an important prognostic factor as to the development of later new occurrences.

The studies by Eisenberg et al., and Althausen et al. suggest that the histological characteristics of the urothelium surrounding noninvasive papillary lesions rather than the histological characteristics of the papillary lesions determine whether or not an invasive lesion will develop. Consequently, at present, careful histological evaluation of the urothelium adjacent to noninvasive papillary lesions and histological study of random biopsies from grossly normal urothelium is the most effective, and perhaps the only practical, predictor of the likelihood of developing invasive bladder carcinoma.

Wolf and Hojgaard's data suggest that this concept extends to superficially invasive tumors. After the removal of a superficially invasive tumor, the fate of the patient is determined by the presence and extent of abnormal changes in the surrounding urothelium.

Red Cell Surface Antigen

The urothelium of the bladder normally has ABH isoantigens on its cell surface, as can be demonstrated by the specific red cell adherence test initially devised by Davidsohn et al. (14). Furthermore, the presence or absence of these surface antigens on noninvasive papillary lesions has been correlated with the propensity of the bladder to develop an invasive lesion. Urothelium that maintains its isoantigens has been shown to be at low risk of developing invasive bladder carcinoma whereas urothelium that has lost its isoantigens is at a high risk of developing invasive bladder carcinoma.

Typical of the results of studies of isoantigens on bladder urothelium is that of Johnson and Lamm (15) who followed 30 patients with initially superficial (Stage O and A) transitional cell bladder tumors. These patients were followed for a minimum of 5 years. Of the 15 patients with negative or absent isoantigens, nine (60%) developed invasive bladder carcinoma. None of the 15 patients who maintained their red cell isoantigens developed invasive bladder carcinoma.

However, those physicians who have attempted to utilize the methods of red cell isoantigens in day-to-day practice are less enthusiastic. Perhaps George Prout (16) at the Massachusetts General Hospital has stated this sense of misgiving most clearly as follows:

> The preoccupation with blood group antigen loss in urothelial tumors continues. Many of us who have tried to use first one technique and then another have not given up but it is certainly difficult to become enthusiastic about a technique that arbitrarily assigns positivity to a specimen if greater than one third of the cells stain with an intensity easily seen on 50X magnification. One wonders if 3 pathologists might not review the hematoxylin and eosin preparations and predict the future for the patient just as well as blood group antigen loss does.

REFERENCES

1. Koss, L. G. (1979): Mapping of the urinary bladder. *Hum. Pathol.*, 10:533–548.
2. Brawn, P. N. (1982): The origin of invasive carcinoma of the bladder. *Cancer*, 50:515–519.
3. Kaye, K. W., and Lange, P. H. (1982): Mode of presentation of invasive bladder carcinoma: reassessment of a problem. *J. Urol.*, 128:31–33.
4. Brawn, P. N. (1983): The relationship between noninvasive papillary lesions and invasive bladder carcinoma. *Cancer*, (In Press).
5. Cohen, S. M., Jacobs, J. B., Arai, M., Johansson, S., and Friedell, G. H. (1976): Early lesions in experimental bladder cancer. 36:2508–2511.
6. Erturk, E., Cohen, S. M., Price, J. M., and Bryant, G. T. (1967): Pathogenesis, histology and transplantability of urinary bladder carcinomas induced in albino rats. *Canc. Res.*, 27:1998–2002.
7. Hicks, R. M., and Wakefield, J. (1972): Rapid induction of bladder cancer in rats with N-methyl-N-nitrourea. I. Histology. *Chem. Biol. Inter.*, 5:139–152.
8. Koss, L. G., and Lavin, P. (1971): Studies of experimental bladder carcinoma in Fischer 344 female rats. *J. Natl. Canc. Inst.*, 46:585–595.

9. Pyrah, L. N., Raper, F. P., and Thomas, G. M. (1964): Report of a follow-up of papillary tumor of the bladder. *Br. J. Urol.*, 36:14–25.

10. Greene, L. F., Hanash, K. A., and Farrow, G. M. (1973): Benign papilloma or papillary carcinoma of the bladder? *J. Urol.*, 110:205–207.

11. Eisenberg, R. B., and Schweinsberg, M. H.: Bladder tumors and associated proliferative mucosal lesions. *J. Urol.*, 84:544–550.

12. Althausen, A. F., Prout, G. R., and Daly, J. D. (1976): Non-invasive papillary carcinoma of the bladder associated with carcinoma in situ. *J. Urol.*, 116:575–580.

13. Wolf, H., and Hojgaard, K. (1983): Prognostic factors in local surgical treatment of invasive bladder cancer with special reference to the presence of urothelial dysplasia. *Cancer*, 51:1710–1715.

14. Davidsohn, I., Kovarik, S., and Lee, C. L. (1966): A, B and H substances in gastrointestinal carcinoma. *Arch. Pathol.*, 81:381–390.

15. Johnson, J. D., and Lamm, D. L. (1980): Prediction of bladder tumor invasion with the mixed cell agglutination test. *J. Urol.*, 123:25–28.

16. Prout, G. R. (1982): Bladder cancer. *J. Urol.*, 128:284.

Chapter 6

Papillomas

PAPILLOMA

Controversy concerning the most appropriate terminology for papillary growths of the urothelium has existed for years. In particular, the papilloma itself occupies the most controversial position, with great variation in its reported frequency. In fact, there have been questions raised about its very existence. Using different criteria to define "papilloma," Mostofi (1) reported only 3% in his series whereas Bergkvist (2) reported a 21% frequency in his series.

The documentation of frequent "recurrences" and the occasional development of invasive carcinoma in a bladder that previously contained a "papilloma" has convinced many pathologists and clinicians that a benign papillary growth either does not exist in the bladder or that if such a benign growth exists, it is extremely rare. Robbins (3) considers papillomas to be "papillary carcinoma, Grade 1" because of their known tendency to recur and become progressively more anaplastic with each recurrence. Pessin and Anderson (4) consider papillomas under the topic of malignant tumors for the following reasons: (a) it is impossible to designate with any degree of certainty which papilloma is benign, (b) more than 50% of so-called papillomas recur, and (c) the great majority of the specimens submitted for diagnosis are biopsies—consequently, the portion of the tumor submitted may not reveal the true picture whereas the deepest part may reveal the malignant character. Kretschmer and Stika (5) recognized that "the pathologist is at a great disadvantage when diagnosing papillary growths because biopsy specimens are frequently inadequate and not representative of the entire tumor. This has led many pathologists to be overly cautious and to call all papillomas malignant—which, of course, is a great injustice to the patient."

Often overlooked is the fact that Meyer Melicow (6) in 1949 concisely evaluated the case of papilloma versus papillary carcinoma in an argument that is only today being fully appreciated:

> I feel keenly that possible chaos may result from the present tendency to drop the term papilloma from the classification of bladder tumors. By benign tumors are meant neoplasms whose component cells are well-differentiated and which contain few mitotic figures, stain evenly and show no evidence of breaking of barriers, and if a bladder tumor reveals such a picture then it is a papilloma regardless of the outcome. By malignant tumors are meant neoplasms whose cellular elements show poor or no differentiation, contain abundant mitotic figures, stain unevenly and give evidence of invasion; and if a bladder tumor shows such a picture it is a carcinoma. Unfortunately, thorough removal of a papilloma does not always result in a cure—patients often have what is called a recurrence. The fault lies not with diagnosing the pathologic condition

or with the histologic criteria of benignity, but with overlooking the fact that though the papilloma was removed the neoplastigenic agent which caused it continues to operate and induces a new tumor (not a recurrence). Another cause for the attempts to discard the term papilloma has been the occasional biopsy specimen that contains only a surface bite of a bladder tumor and appears histologically benign whereas the operative specimen reveals malignant growth. In such a case the tumor was not a papilloma to begin with and the biopsy was not truly representative of the contents. Better and adequate biopsies would eliminate the latter cause.

Friedell (7) has restated the concepts of Melicow as follows:

Often papillomas are relatively small and may be completely removed at the time of cystoscopy. Thus following the complete removal of a superficial papillary lesion from the bladder, the natural history we elucidate through patient follow-up is not the natural history of the lesion we removed, but the natural history of epithelial proliferation elsewhere in the bladder.

Melicow, and later Friedell, clearly understood that the prognosis of patients with papillomas depends primarily on the nature and extent of histological alterations in the urothelium remaining after removal of the benign papilloma. Consequently, pathologists, when examining papillomas, are not being asked to assess the biological potential of the papillomas. Rather, the pathologist is being asked to assess the "malignant potential" of the overall bladder epithelium. This is clearly an impossible task.

Much to their credit, certain physicians, most notably Marshall (8) and Whitmore (9) at the Memorial Sloan Kettering Cancer Center insisted, during a period of time when their point of view was in disfavor, that a benign papillary growth not only exists in the bladder but that its existence is not all that uncommon. They clearly recognized that papillomas rarely, if ever, become invasive and that papillomas have for too long been judged not on their own merits but by the company they keep. A thorough mapping of the urothelium surrounding papillomas demonstrates that papillomas frequently develop in the midst of areas of carcinoma *in situ*, atypical hyperplasia, and simple hyperplasia. Patients with papillomas who develop invasive bladder carcinoma almost invariably develop the invasive bladder carcinoma from the surrounding dysplastic urothelium rather than directly from the preceding papilloma. The finding of a papilloma merely indicates that the adjacent flat urothelium may be in a state of smoldering dysplasia or that the adjacent flat urothelium may already contain areas of malignancy invisible to the naked eye.

Clinical Presentation

Papillomas occur most frequently in the sixth, seventh, and eighth decades of life. Males outnumber females by a ratio of 3:1 to 4:1. The number of patients presenting with a single papilloma is about equal to the number of patients presenting with multiple papillomas. At all ages, in both sexes, painless hematuria is the most common presentation. However, about 15% of patients with papillomas will have severe hematuria (including "clot retention") and 15% will have no history of hematuria at all.

Gross Appearance

Bladder papillomas grow as a complicated fernlike, red, elevated excrescences varying from less than 1 cm to 5 cm in greatest dimension. Fragmentation, necrosis, hemorrhage, and ulceration sometimes distort the usual appearance.

Histology

Bladder papillomas (Figs. 6.1 to 6.18) are composed of delicate papillary fronds, each containing a thin fibrovascular core, covered uniformly by transitional epithelium of variable thickness that generally has a palisaded arrangement. There may be adherence between individual fronds. The papillary epithelium may be slightly and irregularly thickened but without appreciable cellular anaplasia. Mitotic activity may be observed in bladder papillomas but it is generally not prominent. Variable degrees of atypia, consisting of mild cytologic abnormalities and some loss of the usual palisaded arrangement, is present in about one-third of cases.

The base of the papilloma may have pushy margins that extend into the lamina propria and may compress the underlying muscularis. These "pushy margins" are not evidence of invasion.

Location

Melicow (10) recognized that there was a relationship between accumulation and stagnation of urine and the development of papillomas. In dogs, bladder tumors were found to develop in the most dependent portion of the bladder where urine accumulates, i.e., the anterior or inferior wall. In humans, Melicow stated that "most vesical papillomas are located around the trigone and ureteral orifices suggesting that the carcinogenic agent is excreted through the urine and acts with maximum intensity on vulnerable cells in the most dependent portion of the bladder, where the urine accumulates." Due to stagnation of urine, there is a great tendency for bladder tumors, including papillomas, to form within the diverticulum.

Whatever the treatment, further tumors may appear and are found on ever more widely dispersed areas of the bladder urothelium. Although any portion of the bladder may be the site of a papilloma, the anterior bladder wall is the least common site.

Recurrences

The term "recurrence" as employed in this text refers only to the fact that at a later date another tumor was present in the bladder. It does not necessarily mean that a regrowth occurred at the site of a previously removed tumor. Melicow (11) long ago recognized that "recurrences" occurring after complete and careful destruction of preceding tumors were actually new tumors resulting from the continued action of some undefined carcinogenic agent. Operative procedures merely remove the effect and not the cause of papillary growths and the latter continue(s) to act and cause new tumors to form.

Melicow proposed three possible explanations for recurrences:

1. The "recurrences" are regrowths due to inadequate surgery or fulguration.
2. The "recurrences" result from "seeding" or "implants" prior to, during, or after operative procedure.
3. The "recurrences" are new tumors due to the continued action of an unknown carcinogenic agent.

It is obvious that any incompletely removed tumor will continue to grow or "recur." Furthermore, since most operations on the bladder violate the principle of avoidance of direct contact with the cancer field, numerous tumor cells are unavoidably dislodged at surgery. Consequently, occasional "recurrences" have convincingly been shown to result from "seeding" or "implantation" of dislodged tumor cells during the operative procedure. However, the vast majority of "recurrences" appear to be new growths not directly related to the previous tumor(s).

"Recurrences" occur in approximately one-third of patients who initially present with a single papilloma and the recurrence rate increases to approximately 60% in patients who present with multiple papillomas. Patients presenting with multiple papillomas are at a greater risk of subsequently developing invasive bladder carcinoma. This is most likely a reflection that the urothelium surrounding multiple papillomas is likely to have more marked alterations than the urothelium surrounding a single papilloma.

Royce and Spyut (12) studied 68 "recurrences" and found that 43 occurred within 1 year of the diagnosis of the initial tumor, 19 occurred between 1 and 7 years after the diagnosis of the initial tumor, and six occurred between 7 and 15 years after the diagnosis of the initial tumor.

Dedifferentiation

Many studies have shown that a number of "recurrences" or "new occurrences" have a slightly more atypical or dedifferentiated histological appearance than the previously observed lesions. Royce and Spjut (12) found that 7% of their "recurrences" had an increase in grade or malignancy as compared to the original lesions. The Kaiser Foundation (13) studied 92 patients with recurrent papillary lesions and found that 21 progressed to a more advanced grade whereas 71 recurred with the same grade.

A change in grade with "recurrences" should not be unexpected since the "recurrences" are almost invariably new growths, related to the previous papillary lesions only by the fact that they occurred in the same bladder. "Recurrences" that have a more differentiated appearance than the previous lesions are not uncommon.

Prognosis

Royce and Spjut (12) followed 130 consecutive cases of transitional cell tumors they termed "so-called papillomas." These tumors were defined as "containing epithelium normal except that it is usually more cellular. A few normal mitoses may be encountered. Tumor invasion of the subepithelial connective tissue, regardless of the maturity of differentiation, is considered as a higher grade." Nine of the 130 patients were known to have died of carcinoma of the bladder during a follow-up period of 1 to 28 years. Of these nine cases, Royce and Spjut determined that there was:

> ...considerable doubt as to the accuracy of the initial grading of the tumor in most of these nine because of inadequate biopsies. Four of the biopsies, on which the diagnoses were based, were described as "tiny." The other 5 biopsies were taken superficially from tumors of large size. It is very possible that these biopsies did not represent the most malignant parts of the tumor in question.

Royce and Spjut concluded:

> None of the patients who died of carcinoma had an adequate biopsy and there is great doubt that any were actually Grade 1 lesions (so-called papillomas). There is much doubt that any truly Grade 1 lesion (so-called papillomas) behaves as a malignant lesion and the most important part of management is to be certain of the diagnosis.

Whitmore (9) studied 125 patients with bladder papillomas and found that 12 later developed a bladder carcinoma after intervals of 11 months to 20 years. Of these 12 patients, seven (5.5%) had infiltrating carcinomas whereas the remaining five had noninfiltrating carcinoma *in situ*. Whitmore concluded:

> ...the 5 year survival of patients who have only papilloma of the bladder (93.6%) was essentially the same as the 5 year expectancy of the general population of the United States at age 58, whereas the survival of the patients who developed bladder carcinoma was 18.2%, a difference which provides a convincing reason for separating papilloma from bladder carcinoma.

Bergkvist (2) followed 64 cases of papilloma for at least 8 years. None of the patients died of bladder carcinoma, although 11 died of intercurrent disease. The Kaiser Foundation (13) followed 155 patients with papillomas and found that nine (5%) died of bladder carcinoma.

There seems to be a relationship between atypia in a bladder papilloma and a later occurrence of bladder carcinoma. Whitmore (9) found that 33% (12/36) of patients who showed atypism in the initial or recurrent papilloma later developed bladder carcinoma. The increased risk of invasive carcinoma in patients with atypical papillomas may be because of the following: (a) abnormalities in the surrounding urothelium are likely to be more severe in patients with atypical papillomas or (b) the "atypical papillomas" were biopsy specimens that did not reveal the true nature of the lesion, i.e., the deepest part of the atypical papillomas may have been malignant.

The first explanation is more likely since Eisenberg et al. (14) and Althausen et al. (15) have demonstrated that it is not the histological characteristics of the papillomas that determine whether or not an invasive lesion will develop. Rather, the histological characteristics of the surrounding "flat" urothelium is more important. When the surrounding urothelium is normal, the likelihood of developing an invasive lesion is slight whereas the likelihood of developing an invasive lesion increases as abnormalities (atypical hyperplasia, carcinoma *in situ*) appear in the surrounding urothelium. The papillomas appear to be innocent bystanders while, as L. G. Koss (16) has stated, "atypical hyperplasia and carcinoma *in situ* are the common precursors of invasive bladder carcinoma." The finding of a papilloma in the bladder indicates that the entire urothelium, from the renal calyxes to the urethral tip may contain "flat" lesions having an invasive potential. Consequently, a program for regular and continued surveillance of the urinary tract must be planned and executed for the remainder of the patient's life.

Kretschmer and Stika (5) in 1949 emphasized the impact of terminology on the patient by stating:

> Whether or not one is justified in calling all bladder papillomas malignant or potentially malignant is of great importance to the patient, since the patient's entire future depends on this point of view. The patient may contemplate the purchase of new or additional life insurance. Should he be accepted, rejected or "rated up" because he has a papilloma of the bladder, which his physician may consider potentially malignant? The executive who plans to expand his business may hesitate to do so, or stop future contracts, or perhaps retire because he has been told that his papilloma of the bladder is a potentially malignant tumor.

Calling a papilloma cancer will improve one's cure rates but will also add an unnecessary element of terror into the life of the patient. Furthermore, by propagating the concept that papillomas are malignant, attention is detracted from identifying and eradicating the more common precursors of invasive bladder carcinoma, i.e., carcinoma *in situ* and atypical hyperplasia.

INVERTED PAPILLOMA

In 1927 Paschkis (17) described 4 cases of an adenomalike tumor in the bladder. These lesions were discussed in 1954 by Mostofi (18) as an example of the potentialities of bladder epithelium. Potts and Hirst (19) in 1963 designated these tumors as inverted papillomas. These tumors are generally found in the same age range as other papillary lesions of the bladder and have a male-to-female ratio (6:1) that is similar to other papillary lesions of the bladder.

It has been suggested that inverted papillomas may be related to chronic cystitis. Others have noted similarities between inverted papillomas and papillary cystitis, Brunn's nests, cytitis cystica, and cystitis glandularis. It seems likely, however, that inverted papillomas are, as Mostofi determined, an expression of the potentialities of bladder epithelium and are caused by the same etiologic agents that cause other transitional cell tumors, i.e., oncogenic substances, usually unidentified, present in urine.

Symptoms

Symptoms have included the following: (a) symptoms associated with benign prostatic hypertrophy, (b) intermittent urinary retention, (c) macroscopic hematuria, and (d) ureteral colic.

Location

The majority of inverted papillomas have been localized in the trigone, bladder neck, and prostatic urethra. Occasionally, inverted papillomas may occur in the ureter or renal pelvis.

Gross

The lesions have been described as solid, papillary, or pedunculated. The size has ranged up to 7.5 cm in diameter.

Histology

Inverted papillomas (Figs. 6.19 to 6.22) are composed of cords of urothelial-like cells that are inverted and exhibit a mosaic pattern separated by a delicate fibrous stroma. The cords are often cylindrical, creating spaces of varying size that contain a proteinaceous material. The cells are arranged perpendicularly at the periphery, giving a basaloid appearance to the lesion. The surface of the lesion is covered with a urothelium that may be of normal thickness, atrophic, or hyperplastic.

Prognosis

Many investigators have emphasized the benign behavior of inverted papillomas. This belief has been based on the histological appearance of the lesion that lacks nuclear atypia or mitoses and follow-up studies that are usually uneventful. However, Lazarevic and Garret (20) described a case of inverted papilloma associated with a malignant urothelial neoplasm on its surface. They and others have warned against overconfidence in the benign nature of inverted papillomas.

Anderstrom et al. (21) examined nine cases of inverted papillomas and found that two were from bladders that had previously contained bladder tumors. Three of the remaining nine cases developed additional transitional cell tumors following the diagnosis of inverted papilloma, and one of the patients died of metastatic poorly differentiated squamous carcinoma of the bladder. Consequently, it appears that inverted papillomas have the same significance as papillomas of the bladder. Although the inverted papilloma rarely has an invasive capability, the presence of an inverted papilloma indicates that the entire urothelium may be in a state of smoldering dysplasia. Patients with inverted papillomas often have had previous transitional cell tumors and are at an increased risk of developing additional transitional cell tumors. The subsequent tumors, as with simple papillomas, almost invariably develop from the surrounding urothelium and not directly from the preceding inverted papilloma.

REFERENCES

1. Mostofi, F. K. (1960): Standardization of nomenclature and criteria for the diagnosis of epithelial tumors of the urinary bladder. *Acta Un. Int. Cancer*, 16:310–314.
2. Bergkvist, A., Ljungqvist, A., and Moberger, G. (1965): Classification of bladder tumors based on cellular pattern: preliminary report of a clinicopathological study of 300 cases with a minimum follow-up of 8 years. *Acta Chir. Scand.*, 130:371–378.

3. Robbins, S. L. (1967): The lower urinary tract. In: *Pathology*, pp. 1061–1064. W. B. Saunders Co., Philadelphia and London.
4. Pessin, S. B., and Anderson, W. A. D. (1966): Lower urinary tract and male genitalia. In: *Pathology*, 5th ed., edited by W. A. D. Anderson, pp. 663–665. C. V. Mosby Co., St. Louis.
5. Kretschmer, H. L., and Stika, E. (1949): Papilloma of the bladder. *JAMA*, 141:1039–1041.
6. Melicow, M. M. (1949): Discussion of tumors of the bladder. *JAMA*, 141:1047.
7. Friedell, G. H., Bell, J. R., Burney, S. W., Soto, E. A., and Tiltman, A. J. (1976): Histopathology and classification of urinary bladder carcinomas. Urologic Clinics of North America. Vol. 3, No. 1:53–70.
8. Nichols, J. A., and Marshall, V. F. (1956): Treatment of histologically benign papilloma of the urinary bladder by local excision and fulgaration. *Cancer*, 9:566–567.
9. Lerman, R. I., Hutter, R. V., and Whitmore, W. F. (1970): Papilloma of the urinary bladder. *Cancer*, 25:333–342.
10. Melicow, M. M. (1945): Tumors of the urinary drainage tract: urothelial tumors. *J. Urol.*, 186–193.
11. Melicow, M. M. (1952): Histological study of vesical urothelium intervening between gross neoplasms in total cystectomies. *J. Urol.*, 68:261–278.
12. Royce, R. K., and Spjut, H. J. (1959): Transitional cell carcinoma of the bladder, Grade 1 (so-called papilloma). *J. Urol.*, 82:486–489.
13. Gilbert, H. A., Logan, J. L., Kagan, A. R., Friedman, H. A., Cove, J. K., Fox, M., Muldoon, T. M., Lonni, Y. W., Rowe, J. H., Cooper, J. F., Nussbaum, H., Chan, P., Rao, A., and Starr, A. (1978): The natural history of papillary transitional cell carcinoma of the bladder and its treatment in an unselected population on the basis of histologic grading. *J. Urol.*, 119:488–492.
14. Eisenberg, R. B., Roth, R. B., and Schweinsberg, M. H. (1960): Bladder tumors and associated proliferative mucosal lesions. *J. Urol.*, 84:544–550.
15. Althausen, A. F., Prout, G. R., and Daly, J. D. (1976): Non-invasive papillary carcinoma of the bladder associated with carcinoma in situ. *J. Urol.*, 116:575–580.
16. Koss, L. G. (1979): Mapping of the urinary bladder: its impact on the concepts of bladder cancer. *Hum. Pathol.*, 10:533–548.
17. Paschkis, R. (1927): Uber Adenome der Harnblase. *Ztschr. Urol. Chir.*, 21:315.
18. Mostofi, F. K. (1954): Potentialities of bladder epithelium. *J. Urol.*, 71:705–714.
19. Potts, A. F., and Hirst, E. (1963): Inverted papilloma of the bladder. *J. Urol.*, 90:175.
20. Lazarevic, B., and Garret, R. (1978): Inverted papilloma and papillary transitional cell carcinoma of urinary bladder. *Cancer*, 42:1904–1911.
21. Anderstrom, C., Johansson, S., and Pettersson, S. (1982): Inverted papilloma of the urinary tract. *J. Urol.*, 127:1132–1134.

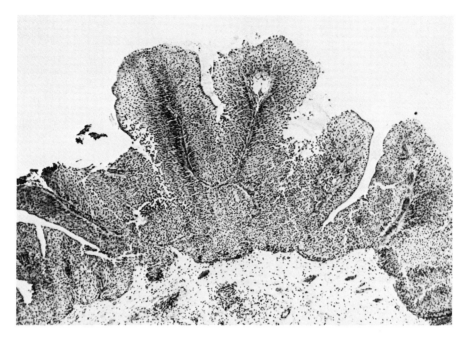

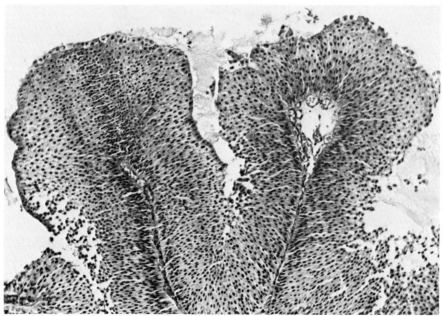

FIGS. 6.1, 6.2. Papilloma. ($\times$40 and $\times$100)

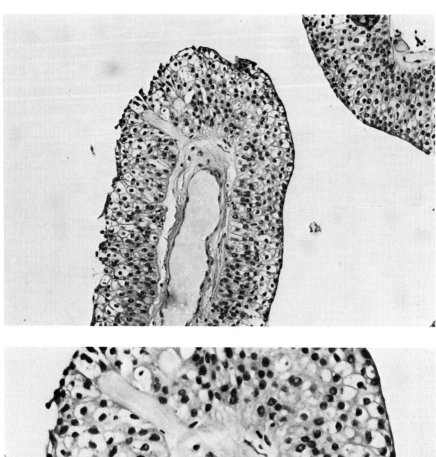

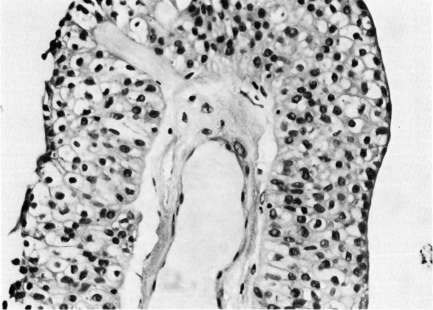

FIGS. 6.3, 6.4.   Papilloma. ($\times 100$ and $\times 200$)

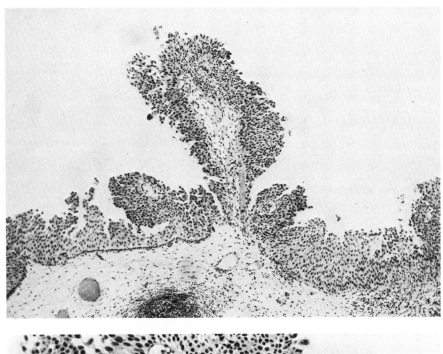

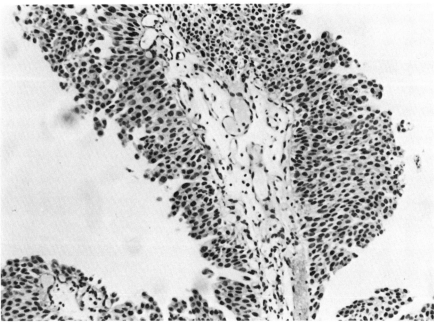

FIGS. 6.5, 6.6. Papilloma. ($\times$40 and $\times$100)

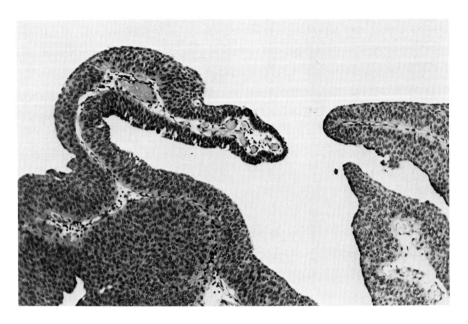

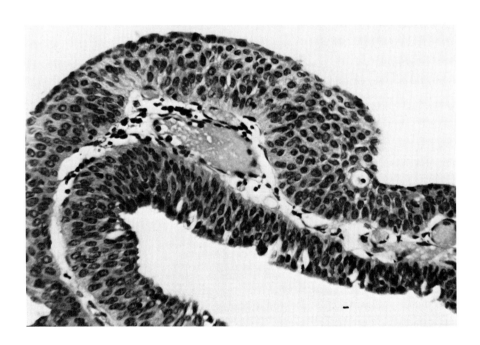

FIGS. 6.7, 6.8.   Papilloma. ($\times$ 40 and $\times$ 100)

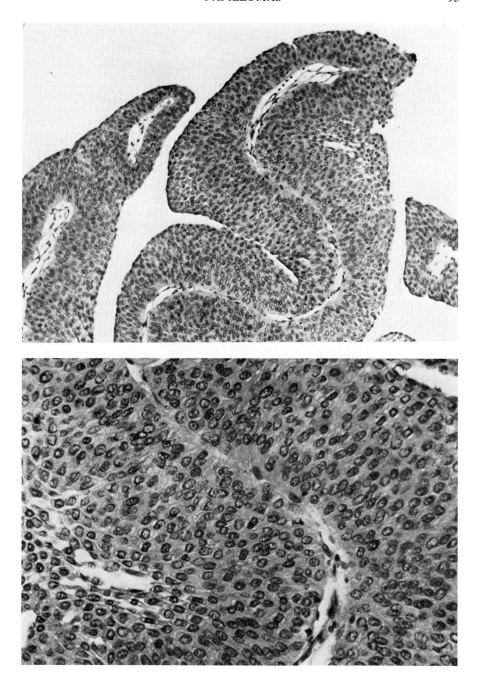

FIGS. 6.9, 6.10. Papilloma. (×40 and ×100)

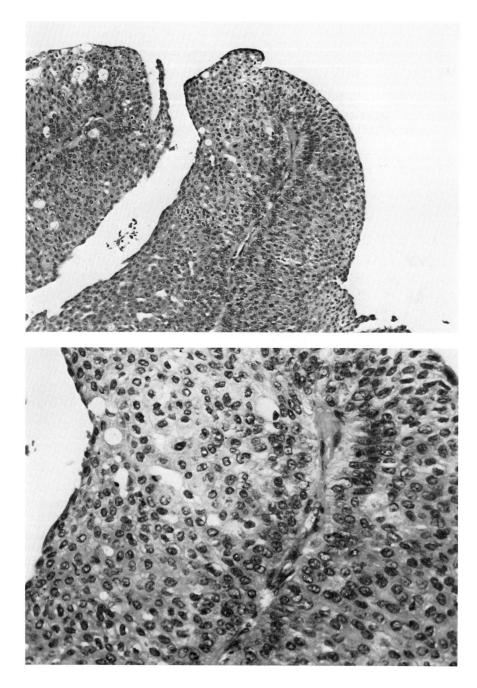

FIGS. 6.11, 6.12.   Papilloma. (×40 and ×100)

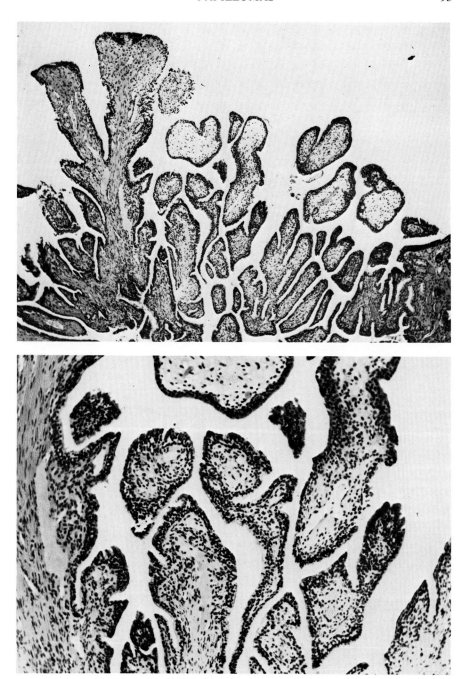

FIGS. 6.13, 6.14. Papilloma. ($\times$40 and $\times$100)

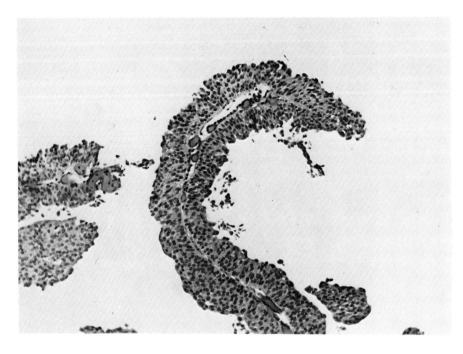

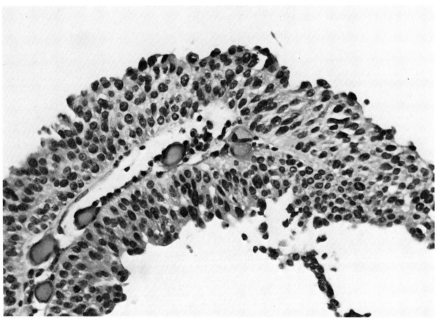

FIGS. 6.15, 6.16. Papilloma. ($\times 40$ and $\times 100$)

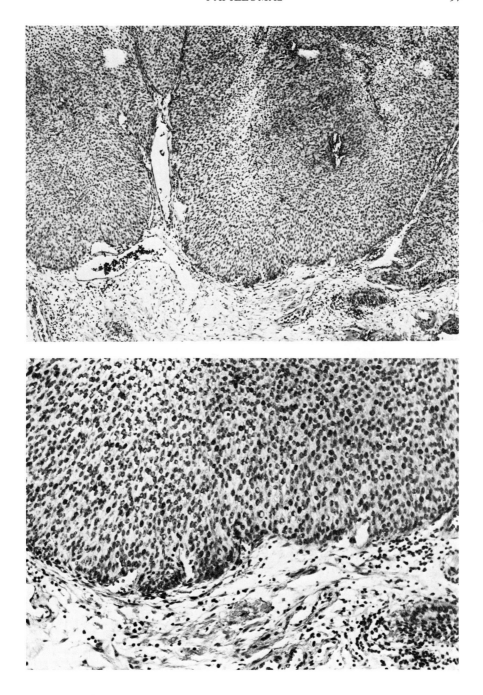

FIGS. 6.17, 6.18. Papilloma showing "pushy margins." (×40 and ×100)

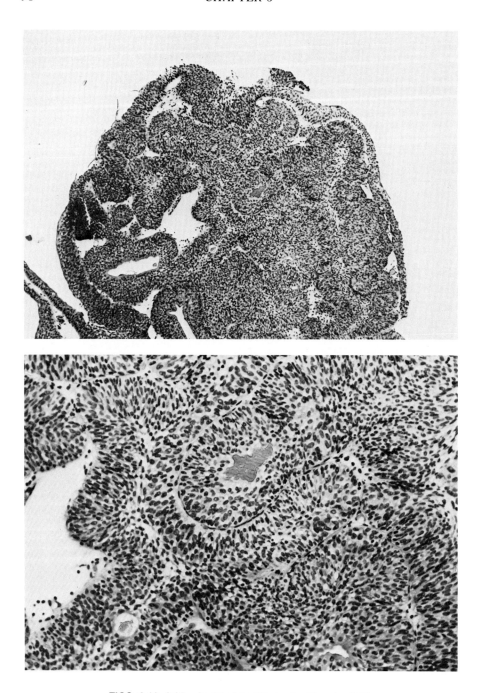

FIGS. 6.19, 6.20.   Inverted papilloma. (×40 and ×100)

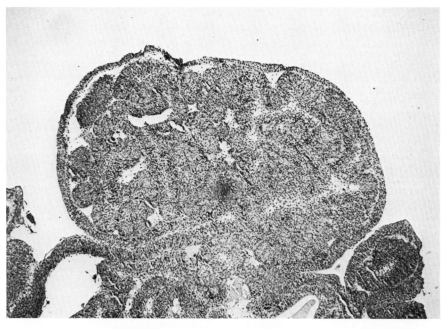

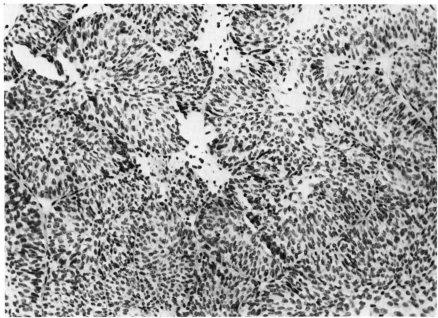

FIGS. 6.21, 6.22. Inverted papilloma. ($\times$40 and $\times$100)

Chapter 7

Papillary Carcinoma

Papillary carcinomas are usually divided into three grades. The distinction among the grades is based on the characteristics of the epithelium. Traditionally, Grade 1 lesions have significant but limited nuclear abnormalities; Grade 2 lesions show significant nuclear abnormalities in about half the cells; and Grade 3 lesions show significant nuclear abnormalities in nearly all the cells (Figs. 7.1 – 7.20).

PAPILLOMA VERSUS NONINVASIVE PAPILLARY CARCINOMA

Pyrah (1) studied 365 cases of papilloma and compared them to 139 cases of noninvasive "early carcinoma." Papillomas were described by Pyrah as:

> Simple tumours with fronded papillae and fine connective tissue cores, covered with transitional epithelium three to five cells thick, regularly arranged with few mitoses. Also included were cases of greater activity in which the number of cell layers was increased, the cells were regularly arranged, mitoses were rare and there was seldom penetration into the stromal cores or subepithelial layer. The pathologist was not prepared to designate these as carcinomata.

"Early carcinoma" was defined by Pyrah as:

> . . . tumours which looked histologically more active and tended to be rather less well-differentiated than papillomas. These tumours were apparently confined to the epithelium without evidence of invasion, but described by the pathologist as being malignant or 'borderline'.

Pyrah followed these cases of noninvasive transitional cell tumors (papillomas and noninvasive "early carcinoma") for at least 5 years and found:

1. In both groups about 70% recur after the first treatment, the recurrences behaving often over many years as benign noninvasive tumours.

2. The death rate from invasive bladder carcinoma in all cases originally designated as papilloma was 6%.

3. The death rate from invasive cancer in all cases originally diagnosed as "early carcinoma" was 7.9%.

Pyrah's study indicates that the prognosis of patients with "papillomas" and patients with noninvasive "early carcinoma" (papillary carcinoma, Grade 1) are similar. Pyrah correctly recognized that neither papillomas or noninvasive "early carcinomas" are common sources of invasive carcinoma by stating:

Thus 6–7% of bladders which at an early stage are the seat of benign papilloma, eventually produce a frankly malignant growth. One of two sequences may occur. One of the recurrent tumours may undergo malignant change or the ultimate malignant tumour may arise at another site in the epithelium. The latter sequence is more likely.

Pyrah and others have recognized that papillomas or papillary carcinomas, Grade 1, are rarely, if ever, invasive. Patients with papillomas or noninvasive papillary carcinomas, Grade 1, may develop invasive bladder carcinoma, but these invasive carcinomas appear to be independent growths unrelated to the previously removed papillary growths. For this reason, it has been suggested that these tumors should be termed "papillary transitional cell tumors" rather than "papillary transitional cell carcinomas."

Gibbons et al. (2) studied 78 patients with single noninvasive papillary transitional cell tumors that were surgically removed. The papillary epithelium was placed into one of four groups: normal, moderate atypia, marked atypia, or carcinoma *in situ*. Those patients whose initial lesions showed normal urothelium, moderate atypia, or marked atypia had approximately the same likelihood of developing an invasive bladder carcinoma, i.e., 20%. However, patients with noninvasive papillary lesions showing carcinoma *in situ* had a 54% chance of developing invasive carcinoma.

Gibbon's data suggests that any person having a noninvasive papillary tumor is at an increased risk of developing invasive carcinoma. The atypia of the noninvasive papillary tumor does not seem to determine whether or not the patient will develop invasive carcinoma since papillary tumors with normal urothelium, and urothelium showing moderate and marked atypia, had the same incidence of subsequently developing invasive lesions. Furthermore, since these noninvasive lesions are presumably amenable to surgical removal, no cells should remain after excision to propagate further growths. More likely, it is the atypia present in the surrounding urothelium that determines whether or not an invasive lesion will develop.

Gibbon's study indicates that patients with noninvasive papillary tumors with epithelium showing changes that have progressed past atypia to carcinoma *in situ* are at a markedly increased risk of developing invasive carcinoma. This may indicate that (a) patients with noninvasive papillary lesions with carcinoma *in situ* are at an increased risk of having severe abnormalities in the surrounding urothelium or (b) noninvasive papillary lesions with areas of carcinoma *in situ* are more likely to have areas of invasion that were undetected in the biopsy specimen.

It is likely that the first hypothesis is correct in most cases. Following the complete removal of a noninvasive papillary lesion with focal carcinoma *in situ* the natural history we elicit through follow-up studies is the natural history of the surrounding urothelium. The urothelium surrounding noninvasive papillary lesions with focal carcinoma *in situ* is likely to contain severe abnormalities capable of invasion. Even if the papillary lesion has undetected areas of invasion, Wolf and Hojgaard (3) have shown that after complete removal of superficially invasive lesions the histology of the surrounding urothelium, not the histology of the superficially invasive lesions, determines whether or not additional tumors will develop.

RELATIONSHIP BETWEEN NONINVASIVE TRANSITIONAL CELL TUMORS AND SUBSEQUENT INVASIVE LESIONS

Numerous studies have demonstrated that the epithelial atypia of the completely removed noninvasive papillary transitional cell tumor does not determine whether or not an invasive lesion will develop. Rather, the histological changes in the urothelium surrounding the noninvasive lesions are of more importance. Althausen (4) evaluated 129 patients with low grade, low stage transitional cell tumors with a minimum follow-up of 5 years. Seventy-eight of the 129 patients had sufficient urothelium adjacent to the transitional cell tumor for study. Althausen et al. found that:

1. Forty-one of the 78 cases had normal urothelium adjacent to the transitional cell tumor. Three of these 41 cases (7%) developed an invasive bladder carcinoma.

2. Twenty-five of the 78 cases had atypical urothelium adjacent to the transitional cell tumor. Nine of these 25 cases (36%) developed an invasive bladder carcinoma.

3. Twelve of the 78 cases had carcinoma *in situ* in the urothelium adjacent the transitional cell tumor. Ten of these 12 cases (83%) developed an invasive bladder carcinoma.

Eisenberg (5) has shown that the likelihood of invasive carcinoma occurring following a noninvasive papillary lesion was largely determined by the surrounding urothelium. In Eisenberg's study, eight patients had no additional tumors following the removal of a noninvasive papillary lesion. These eight patients all had normal urothelium adjacent to the papillary lesions. Seven patients developed fatal invasive carcinomas following the removal of a noninvasive papillary lesion. These seven cases all had proliferative lesions (hyperplasia or carcinoma *in situ*) in the urothelium surrounding the papillary lesions.

The studies of Eisenberg et al. and Althausen et al. both indicate that the likelihood of invasive carcinoma developing in patients with noninvasive papillary lesions is determined not by the histological characteristics of the papillary lesion but by the histological characteristics of the surrounding urothelium. The surrounding urothelium may contain areas of carcinoma *in situ* or atypical hyperplasia that appear to be the more common precursors to invasive bladder carcinoma.

The dominant role of the surrounding urothelium extends to superficially invasive bladder tumors (invasion of lamina propria or superficial muscle). Wolf and Hojgaard (3) studied 25 patients with such lesions and found that when the surrounding urothelium was normal, recurrent lesions developed in only two of 17 cases whereas recurrent lesions developed in seven of eight cases that had dysplasia or carcinoma *in situ* in the surrounding urothelium.

IMPORTANCE OF INVASION AND GRADING

While Grade 1 papillary carcinomas are rarely invasive, Grade 2 and Grade 3 lesions are more likely to be intimately associated with an invasive lesion. Whether these invasive lesions develop directly from the papillary tumors or develop in surrounding "flat" urothelium and secondarily involve the papillary tumor is not always clear.

Marshall (6) has shown that there is a correlation between grade and stage. Low grade bladder tumors are usually low stage tumors whereas high grade bladder tumors are likely to be at a more advanced stage. Of the two entities, the presence or absence of invasion is probably more important than the grade of the tumor. This was demonstrated by Bergkvist et al. who studied 104 Grade 2 papillary carcinomas. Bergkvist defined Grade 2 papillary carcinomas as:

> ... the papillary epithelium is thickened and displays moderate cellular deviation with some variation in the size of the cells and nuclei. A tendency to loose the normal polarity of individual cells is also noted.

Bergkvist (7) followed these 104 cases for up to 8 years. Twenty of the 104 cases died of causes other than bladder carcinoma. Of the remaining 84 cases, 15 showed no invasion, 33 had obvious invasion, and in 36 cases invasion was suspected but not definitely demonstrated. The 15 cases showing no invasion all survived 8 years whereas 29 of the 33 cases showing obvious invasion died of bladder carcinoma within 8 years, and 25 of the 36 cases with suspected invasion died of bladder carcinoma within 8 years.

In a study of 2,634 patients with bladder carcinoma, Mostofi (8) demonstrated that survival correlates with both the grade of the tumor and the presence or absence of invasion. Mostofi followed these patients for 12 years and found:

Expected Survival	70%
Papillary, Grade 1, no invasion	60%
Papillary, Grade 2, no invasion	42%
Papillary, Grade 2, invasion	25%
Papillary, Grade 3, invasion	15%
Infiltrating, Grade 2 and 3	9%

The studies of Bergkvist and Mostofi emphasize that it is essential that the pathology report clearly state the presence or absence of invasion. If invasion is not subject to evaluation due to fragmentation, small sample size, or tissue distortion, this should be noted.

REFERENCES

1. Pyrah, L. N., Raper, F. P., and Thomas, G. M. (1964): Report of a follow-up of papillary tumours of the bladder. *Br. J. Urol.*, 36:14–25.
2. Gibbons, R. P., Mandler, J. I., and Hartmann, W. H. (1969): The significance of epithelial atypia seen in non-invasive transitional cell papillary tumors of the bladder. *J. Urol.*, 102:195–199.
3. Wolf, H., and Hojgaard, K. (1983): Prognostic factors in local surgical treatment of invasive bladder cancer with special reference to the presence of urothelial dysplasia. *Cancer*, 51:1710–1715.
4. Althausen, A. F., Prout, G. R., and Daly, J. D. (1976): Non-invasive papillary carcinoma of the bladder associated with carcinoma in situ. *J. Urol.*, 116:575–580.
5. Eisenberg, R. B., Roth, R. B., and Schweinsberg, M. H. (1960): Bladder tumors and associated proliferative mucosal lesions. *J. Urol.*, 84:544–550.

6. Marshall, V. F. (1952): The relation of the preoperative estimate to the pathologic demonstration of the extent of vesical neoplasms. *J. Urol.*, 68:714–723.
7. Bergkvist, A., Ljungqvist, A., and Moberger, G. (1965): Classification of bladder tumors based on cellular pattern: preliminary report of a clinicopathological study of 300 cases with a minimum follow-up of 8 years. *Acta Chir. Scand.*, 130:371–378.
8. Mostofi, F. K. (1956): A study of 2678 patients with initial carcinoma of the bladder: I. Survival rates. *J. Urol.*, 75:480–491.

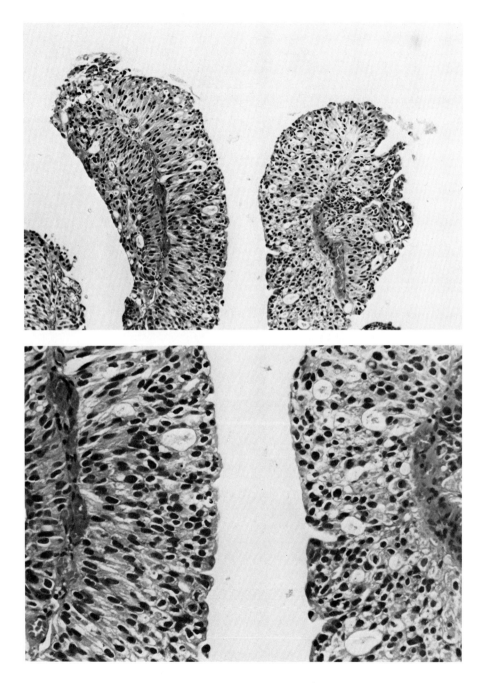

FIGS. 7.1, 7.2. Papillary transitional cell carcinoma, Grade 1. ($\times 40$ and $\times 100$)

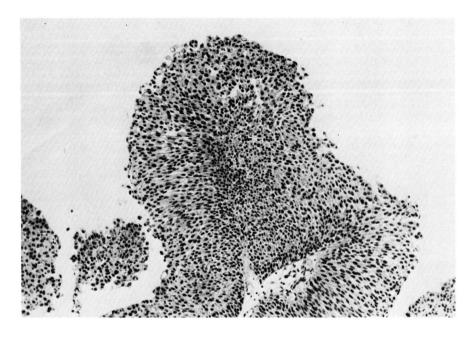

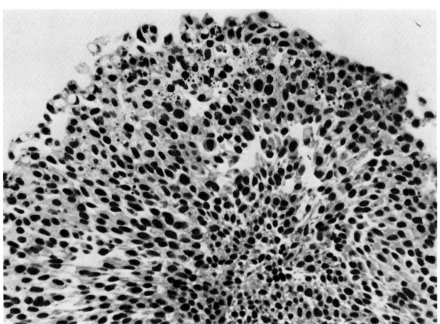

FIGS. 7.3, 7.4. Papillary transitional cell carcinoma, Grade 1. ($\times$40 and $\times$100)

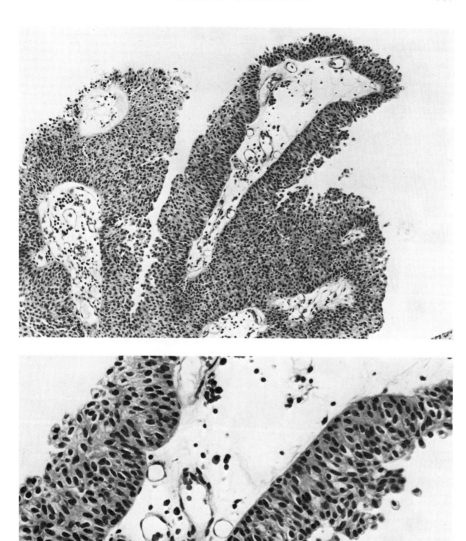

FIGS. 7.5, 7.6. Papillary transitional cell carcinoma, Grade 1. (×40 and ×100)

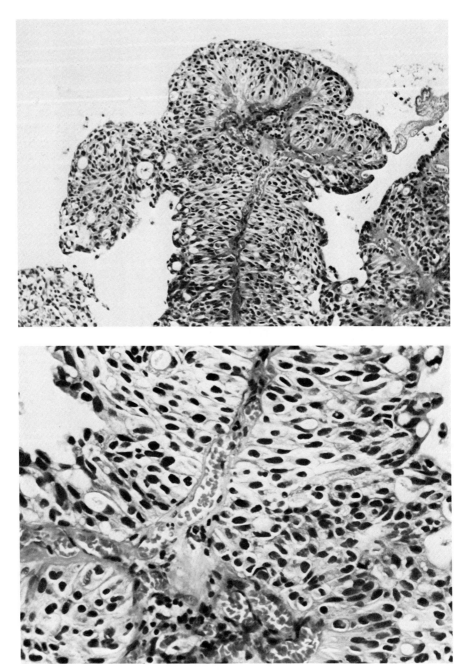

FIGS. 7.7, 7.8. Papillary transitional cell carcinoma, Grade 2. ($\times$40 and $\times$100)

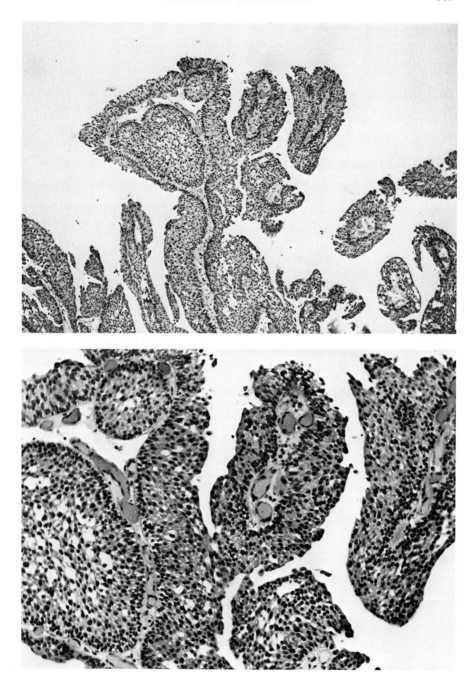

FIGS. 7.9, 7.10. Papillary transitional cell carcinoma, Grade 2. (×40 and ×100)

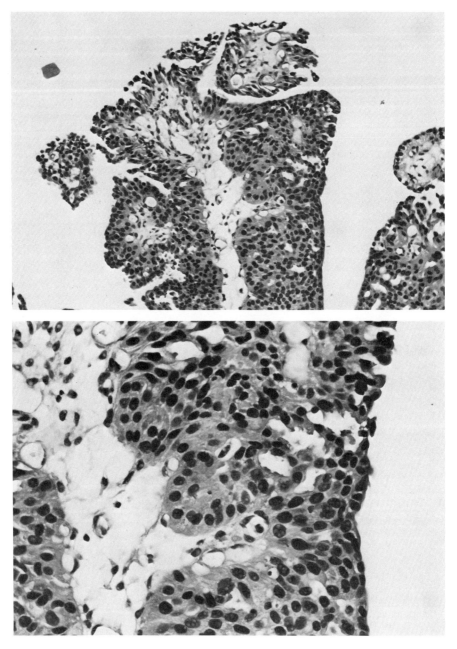

FIGS. 7.11, 7.12. Papillary transitional cell carcinoma, Grade 2. ($\times 40$ and $\times 100$)

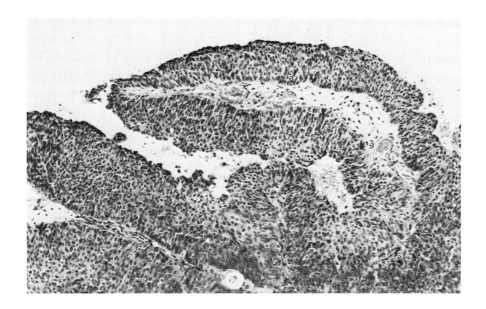

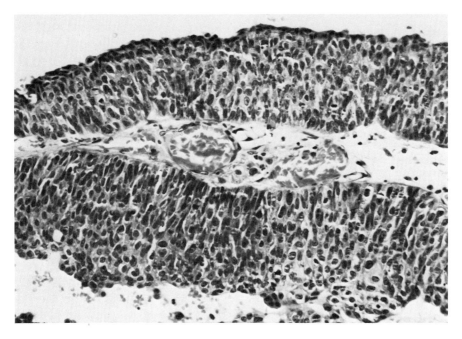

FIGS. 7.13, 7.14. Papillary transitional cell carcinoma, Grade 3. ($\times$40 and $\times$100)

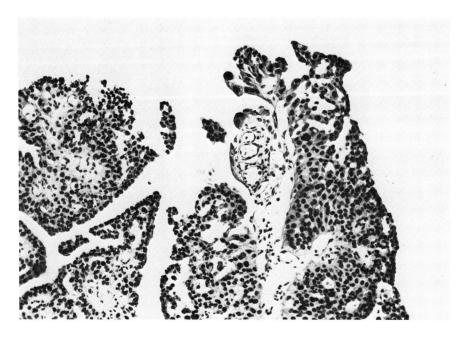

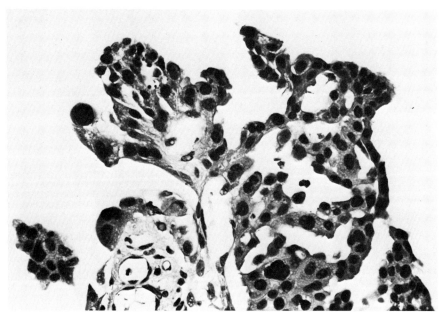

FIGS. 7.15, 7.16. Papillary transitional cell carcinoma, Grade 3. ($\times 40$ and $\times 100$)

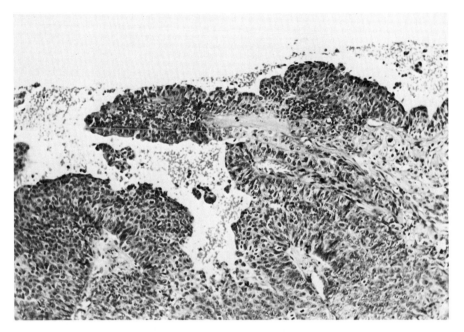

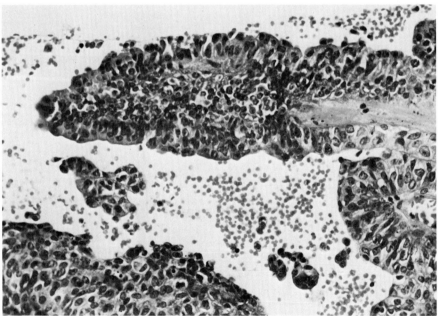

FIGS. 7.17, 7.18. Papillary transitional cell carcinoma, Grade 3. (×40 and ×100)

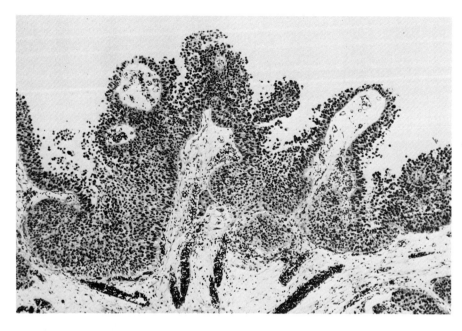

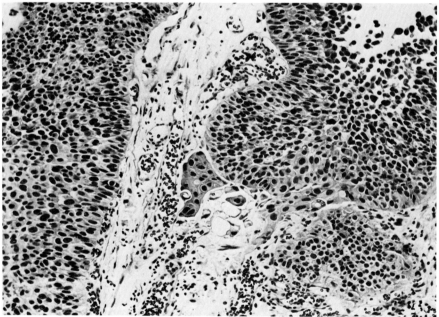

FIGS. 7.19, 7.20. Papillary transitional cell carcinoma showing focal invasion of lamina propria. (×40 and ×100)

Chapter 8

Carcinoma *In Situ*

The discovery of carcinoma *in situ* of the urinary system was almost accidental. In seeking to explain the frequent "recurrences" of bladder cancer, Meyer Melicow (1) in 1952 studied 10 bladder specimens, all containing invasive bladder carcinoma. Sections of the grossly obvious invasive bladder carcinoma as well as sections from normal-appearing urothelium surrounding the bladder tumor were studied. The normal-appearing urothelium surrounding the invasive carcinomas contained not only areas of inflammation, urothelial hyperplasia, and metaplasia, but also contained occasional areas of pronounced cellular atypia that Melicow designated as carcinoma *in situ*. Melicow concluded that adjacent to grossly obvious bladder tumor there may be present, unseen by the naked eye, focal areas of cancerous change that in time come of age and become grossly appreciated and clinically obvious.

In another report, also in 1952, Melicow and Hollowell (2) presented a more definitive study of carcinoma *in situ* of the bladder. Melicow and Hollowell demonstrated that carcinoma *in situ* can occur in any portion of the urothelium, from the kidney to the urethra, and they stressed that carcinoma *in situ* of the bladder are clinically deceptive lesions, malignant from their onset, that can be highly invasive and that only early adequate eradication can hold a promise of a cure.

The existence of carcinoma *in situ*, as described by Melicow, was soon supported by urine cytology studies. Crabbe (3) in 1956 found cancer cells in the urine of dyestuff workers prior to the appearance of a tumor. Melamed (4) in 1960 noted a latent period between the finding of urine cytology containing malignant cells and the discovery of a visible focus of carcinoma *in situ*. The malignant cells observed by both Melamed and Crabbe presumably were derived from grossly normal bladder urothelium that, unseen by the naked eye, contained areas of carcinoma *in situ*.

Other studies confirmed Melicow's suggestion that, unseen by the naked eye, urothelium adjacent to gross bladder tumor frequently contained areas of atypia and carcinoma *in situ*. Eisenberg et al. (5) found proliferative lesions adjacent to 26% of noninvasive papillary lesions and adjacent to 60% of invasive tumors. Simon, Cordonnier, et al. (6) found "proliferative mucosal change" in 34 of 38 cystectomy cases and noted that the "proliferative mucosal changes" were most frequently found in close proximity to the primary tumor. Schade and Swinney (7,8) studied multiple biopsy specimens from 100 patients with bladder carcinoma and found "atypia" in 86% of the cases. This "atypia" was severe enough in 40% of cases to warrant a diagnosis of carcinoma *in situ*. Cooper et al. (9) and Skinner et al. (10) found "severe epithelial atypia" adjacent to the primary neoplasm in 42 to 100% of the cases and found "severe epithelial atypia" in 33 to 55% of the cases at a site distant from the papillary neoplasm. They found that the likelihood of urothelial abnormalities increased as the primary bladder neoplasm became more poorly differentiated. Friedell (11) and Koss (12) embedded entire bladder specimens and observed a high incidence of urothelial abnormalities in bladders with a primary neoplasm. They noted that patients with recurrent or multiple tumors had the most marked and widespread changes.

Other studies have documented that the urothelial changes in a patient with a bladder tumor are not limited to the bladder. Schade and Swinney (7,8) found that 33% of patients with bladder tumors had carcinoma *in situ* in the ureter. Other studies have shown that patients with bladder tumors are at an increased risk of having carcinoma *in situ* of the renal pelvis or urethra.

The continuing studies of Koss, Melamed et al. (13) of 503 men accidentally exposed to para-aminophenone compounds has supplied much of our clinical knowledge of the development of carcinoma *in situ* and invasive carcinoma following exposure to carcinogens. In that group of men, 35 have developed invasive bladder carcinoma and an additional 13 have developed carcinoma *in situ*. Of the 13 men with carcinoma *in situ*, seven have subsequently developed invasive carcinoma. The location and histology of the tumors were similar to bladder tumors developing without known carcinogenic stimulation.

SYMPTOMS

There are few specific symptoms that can aid in the clinical diagnosis of carcinoma *in situ*. However, at least 90% of patients with carcinoma *in situ* of the bladder have symptoms of frequency, dysuria, urgency, and gross or microscopic hematuria.

Remission of clinical symptoms and cystoscopic abnormalities occasionally occur spontaneously. However, the symptoms usually persist and are apparent long before the tumor is recognized cystoscopically. In a study at the Mayo Clinic, (14) the average symptomatic period between onset of symptoms and discovery of cytological abnormalities in the urine was 32 months. There appeared to be a direct relationship between the intensity of the symptoms and the invasiveness of the tumor. Also at the Mayo Clinic, (15) in a review of 486 patients treated for interstitial cystitis during a 10-year period, carcinoma *in situ* of the bladder was ultimately identified in 23% of men and 1.3% of women. The Mayo Clinic study concluded that all patients, especially males, who have unexplained, unrelenting, or recurrrent lower urinary tract symptoms, irrespective of the presence or absence of bacteruria, should have urinary cytologic and cystoscopic examinations.

GROSS

Findings at cystoscopy depend on the stage of development. In its inception, carcinoma *in situ* appears to affect the subsurface cells that do not cause visible alterations to the urothelium. When the process extends to include the surface cells, the urothelium may appear reddish or yellowish with a granular or cobblestone appearance. The lesions rarely have a well-defined border since carcinoma *in situ* usually merges with areas of inflammation and atypia. Vascular proliferation may cause the urothelium to appear soft and red on cystoscopic examination. Urothelial invaginations, such as Brunn's nests, may appear as "yellow dots" and carcinoma *in situ* may extend into these invaginations. It is impossible to tell if normal-appearing mucosa is really free of carcinoma *in situ*.

Carcinoma *in situ* most commonly occurs adjacent to an obvious exophytic tumor. Other sites of predilection correspond with the known distribution of invasive carcinoma, i.e., base of the bladder, trigone, ureteral orifices, posterior and lateral walls. Carcinoma *in situ* is rare in the anterior wall or dome of the bladder.

HISTOLOGY

The urothelium of carcinoma *in situ* (Figs. 8.1–8.12) varies in thickness from one cell to a thickness of 10 to 20 cells. The surface of the urothelium may be irregular, and the cells of the urothelium contain the classic criteria of malignancy, i.e., nuclear enlargement, hyperchromatism, irregularity, and nucleolar prominence. The cells may be monotonously similar or bizarrely different. The increased size of the nuclei coupled with a reduced amount of cytoplasm creates an impression of crowding. The loss of the usual sequential maturation and the loss of individual cell polarity creates a disorganized or disorderly appearance. Mitoses may not only be common but may be abnormal.

The histological changes of carcinoma *in situ* may blend with areas of atypical hyperplasia. This finding suggests that there is a gradual and progressive transition of premalignant atypia into carcinoma *in situ*. The diagnosis of carcinoma *in situ* versus severe dysplasia is often subjective, depending on the experience of the pathologist who must make a qualitative and quantitative assessment of a variety of histological features. Meyer Melicow, taking into account the subjective nature of a diagnosis of carcinoma *in situ* has admonished that the danger is now "over-diagnosis" (16).

DIAGNOSIS

The most valuable test for screening, diagnosis, and follow-up of carcinoma *in situ* is an accurately conducted and interpreted cytologic examination. Almost all carcinomas *in situ* exhibit anaplastic, Grade 3 or 4, morphologic alterations, with a loss of intercellular cohesiveness. These alterations enhance the suitability of detecting carcinoma *in situ* through cytological studies. In one series, all of the carcinomas *in situ* were detected through cytological examination (14).

Random biopsies of apparently normal urothelium taken at the time of removal of superficial bladder tumors are a common source of carcinoma *in situ*. Studies of this phenomenon have demonstrated that patients with noninvasive papillary growths or patients with superficially invasive tumors have an ominous prognosis when the surrounding urothelium contains areas of carcinoma *in situ*.

PROGNOSIS

Since Melicow's discovery of carcinoma *in situ* in 1952, there has been increasing speculation that carcinoma *in situ* is a common source of invasive bladder carcinoma. In fact, L. G. Koss (17) has stated that "atypical hyperplasia and carcinoma *in situ* are the common source of invasive bladder carcinoma." Although the appearance of carcinoma *in situ* as a "pure" phenomenon is being recognized with increasing frequency, it is well recognized that carcinoma *in situ* is difficult to detect and study in a pure state. To date, most cases of carcinoma *in situ* have been detected adjacent to grossly evident bladder tumors. The natural history elicited through follow-up of these cases may not reflect the natural history of pure carcinoma *in situ*.

Melamed (18) followed 25 patients with carcinoma *in situ*. The diagnosis of carcinoma *in situ* was based on biopsy or operative specimens. As well as could be determined, none of the 25 patients had invasive carcinoma at the time of the initial diagnosis of carcinoma *in situ*. Of these patients:

1. Eight had radical cystectomies shortly after the diagnosis of carcinoma *in situ*. None of these patients developed disseminated bladder carcinoma.

2. Six were treated by nonsurgical means. These patients were free of invasive carcinoma 1 month to 5 years after the diagnosis of carcinoma *in situ*.

3. Nine developed invasive bladder carcinoma after intervals ranging from 8 to 67 months.

4. Two developed metastatic bladder carcinoma.

Utz et al. (19) at the Mayo Clinic followed 62 cases of carcinoma *in situ*. These cases were pure without concomitant invasion or papillary lesions. Initial treatment in 56 patients consisted of cystoscopic biopsy with transurethral electroresection and fulguration. Radiotherapy was administered in two patients. The bladder was removed in three cases. One patient had a segmental resection. Of these patients:

1. Thirty-seven developed invasive bladder carcinoma that was fatal in 24 cases.

2. Twenty-five did not develop invasive bladder carcinoma (two had persistent carcinoma *in situ*, 18 were apparently well at the end of the study, and five died of unrelated causes).

In both the study by Melamed et al. (18) and the study by Utz et al. (19), additional cases of invasive carcinoma may have developed had the follow-up period been extended.

Theoretically, since carcinoma *in situ* is limited to the urothelium without invasion of the underlying tissue, these lesions should be cured by total cystectomy. Farrow et al. (14) studied 21 cases of early bladder carcinoma that were detected by cytology and treated by total cystectomy. The neoplasms were entirely *in situ* in 17 of the 21 patients whereas four of the tumors showed minimal microinvasion in addition to carcinoma *in situ*. None of the patients at the conclusion of the study had developed metastatic bladder carcinoma. However, it is well known that patients with carcinoma *in situ* of the bladder are at an increased risk of having similar changes in the urethra or ureters. After total cystectomy, an invasive lesion could develop from the urothelium of the urethra or ureters. In one series, three of 13 (10) cystectomized patients in whose distal ureter CIS was found suffered subsequent transitional cell carcinoma in the upper collecting system necessitating nephroureterectomy, whereas in another series, (20) one of seven patients with ureteral CIS at cystectomy performed for bladder cancer developed an invasive ureteral tumor necessitating nephroureterectomy 31 months later, and in a third study, five of seven patients with CIS of the bladder (21) displayed like lesions in the prostatic urethra and ducts with invasive transitional cell carcinoma spreading to involve the seminal vesicles in one instance.

It is possible that spontaneous regression of carcinoma *in situ* may occur if the carcinogenic agent is eliminated and the patient has adequate immune defenses. However, most studies indicate that there is a steady progression to invasiveness. Farrow at the Mayo Clinic (14), Koss et al. (12) and Skinner et al. (10) have demonstrated that invasive bladder cancer occurs only after there are widespread areas of carcinoma *in situ* or mucosal atypia. In the Mayo Clinic study, only 4 of 21 cases of carcinoma *in situ* showed microinvasion despite the fact that 15 of 21 patients had CIS involving more than one-third of the mucosa examined and 9 patients had CIS involving over 50% of the mucosa examined.

It appears that carcinoma *in situ* of the bladder is increasing in frequency. The increase in frequency is probably due to three factors: (a) an actual increase due to increased exposure to industrial oncogens, food additives, etc.; (b) a relative increase due to greater awareness by urologists as to the possible presence of carcinoma *in situ*; and (c) improvement in techniques, particularly cytological preparation and interpretation, necessary to diagnose cases of carcinoma *in situ*.

REFERENCES

1. Melicow, M. M. (1952): Histological study of vesical urothelium intervening between gross neoplasms in total cystectomy. *J. Urol.*, 68:261–278.
2. Melicow, M. M., and Hollowell, J. W. (1952): Intra-urothelial cancer: carcinoma in situ. Bowen's disease of the urinary system. Discussion of thirty cases. *J. Urol.*, 68:763–772.
3. Crabbe, J. C., Cresdee, W. C., and Scott, T. S. (1956): The cytological diagnosis of bladder tumor amongst dyestuff workers. *Br. J. Ind. Med.*, 13:270–276.
4. Melamed, M. R., Koss, L. G., Ricci, A., and Whitmore, W. F. (1960): Cytohistological observations on developing carcinoma of urinary bladder in man. *Cancer*, 13:67–74.
5. Eisenberg, R. B., Roth, R. B., and Schweinsberg, M. H. (1960): Bladder tumors and associated proliferative mucosal lesions. *J. Urol.*, 84:544–550.
6. Simon, W., Cordonnier, J. J., Snodgrass, W. T. (1962): Pathogenesis of bladder carcinoma. *J. Urol.*, 88:797–802.
7. Schade, R. O. K., and Swinney, J. (1968): Precancerous changes in bladder epithelium. *Lancet*, 2:943–946.
8. Schade, R. O. K., and Swinney, J. (1973): The association of urothelial atypism with neoplasia: its importance in treatment and prognosis. *J. Urol.*, 109:619–622.
9. Cooper, P. H., Waisman, J., Johnson, W. H., and Skinner, D. G. (1973): Severe atypia of transitional epithelium and carcinoma of the urinary bladder. *Cancer*, 31:1055–1060.
10. Skinner, D. G., Richie, J. R., Cooper, P. H., Waisman, J., and Kaufman, J. J. (1974): The clinical significance of carcinoma in situ of the bladder and its association with overt carcinoma. *J. Urol.*, 112:68–71.
11. Austen, G. J., and Friedell, G. H. (1964): Observations on local growth patterns of bladder cancer. *Trans. Am. Assoc. Genit. Surg.*, 56:38–43.

12. Koss, L. G., Tiamson, E. M., and Robbins, M. A. (1974): Mapping cancerous and precancerous bladder changes. A study of urothelium in ten surgically removed bladders. *JAMA*, 227:281–286.
13. Koss, L. G., Melamed, M. R., and Kelly, R. E. (1969): Further cytologic and histologic studies of bladder lesions in workers exposed to para-aminodiphenyl. *J. Natl. Cancer Inst.*, 43:233–243.
14. Farrow, G. M., Utz, D. C., and Rife, C. C. (1976): Morphological and clinical observations of patients with early bladder cancer treated with total cystectomy. *Cancer Res.*, 36:2495–2501.
15. Utz, D. C., and Zincke, H. (1974): The masquerade of bladder cancer in situ as interstitial cystitis. *J. Urol.*, 111:160–161.
16. Melicow, M. M. (1976): Carcinoma in situ: an historical prospective. *Urol. Clin. North Am.*, Feb., Vol. 3, No. 1:5–11.
17. Koss, L. G. (1979): Mapping of the urinary bladder. *Hum. Pathol.*, 10:533–548.
18. Melamed, M. R., Voutsa, N. G., and Grabstald, H. (1964): Natural history and clinical behavior of in situ carcinoma of the human urinary bladder. *Cancer*, 17:1533–1545.
19. Utz, D. C., Hanash, K. A., Farrow, G. M. (1970): The plight of the patient with carcinoma in situ of the bladder. *J. Urol.*, 103:160–164.
20. Linker, D. G., and Whitmore, W. F. (1975): Ureteral carcinoma in situ. *J. Urol.*, 113:777–780.
21. Seemayer, T. A., Knaack, J., Thelmo, W. L., Wang, N. S., and Ahmed, M. N. (1975): Further observations on carcinoma in situ of the urinary bladder: silent but extensive intraprostatic involvement. *Cancer*, 36:514–520.

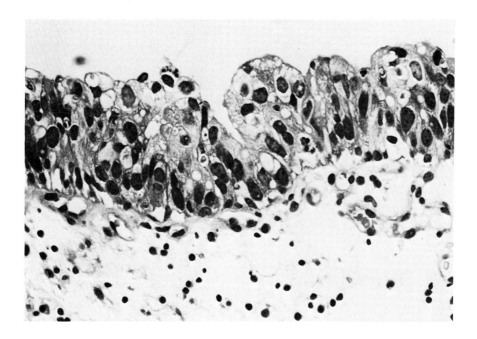

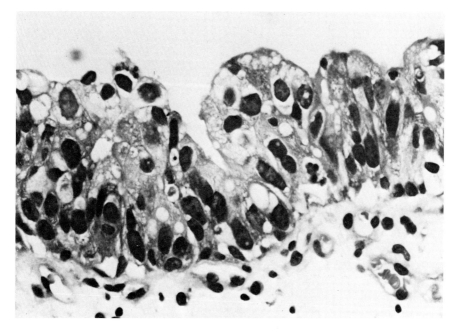

FIGS. 8.1, 8.2. Carcinoma *in situ*. (×100 and ×200)

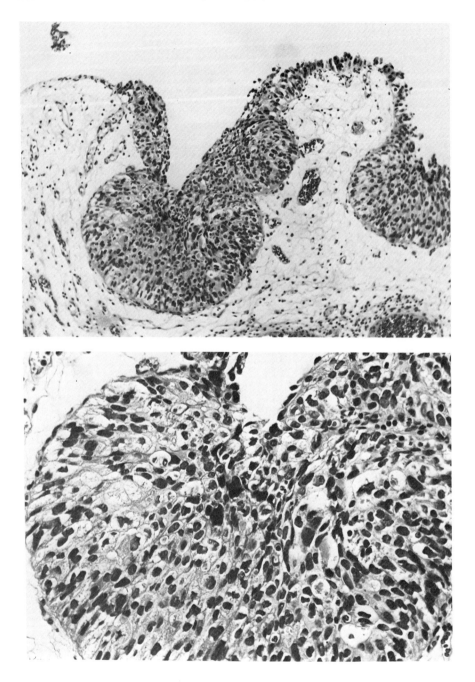

FIGS. 8.3, 8.4. Carcinoma *in situ.* ($\times$100 and $\times$200)

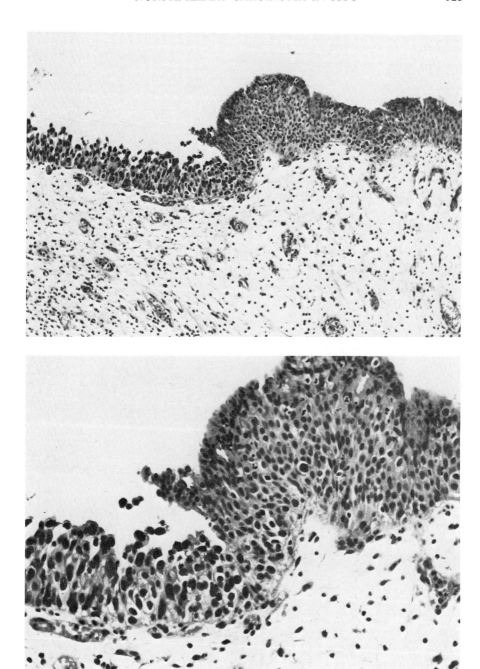

FIGS. 8.5, 8.6. Carcinoma *in situ (left)* adjacent atypical hyperplasia *(right).* (×100 and ×200)

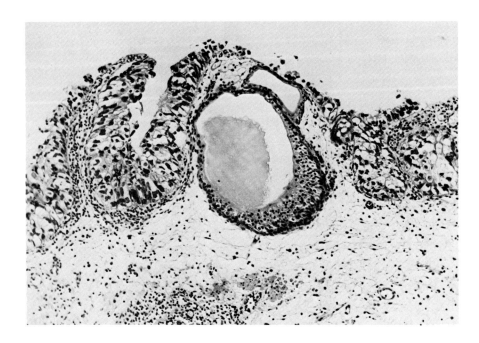

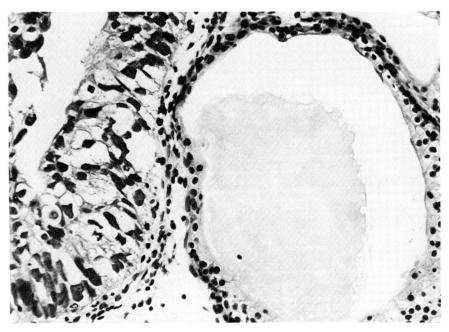

FIGS. 8.7, 8.8.   Carcinoma *in situ.* (×100 and ×200)

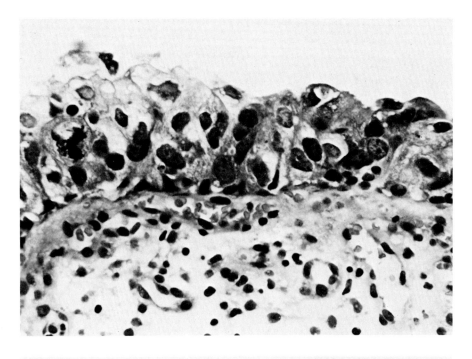

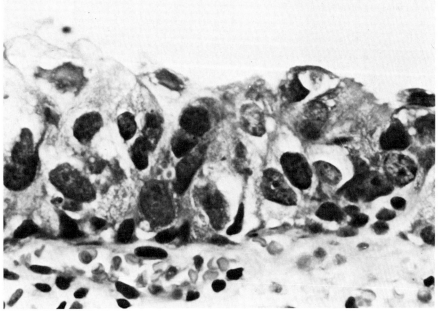

FIGS. 8.9, 8.10.   Carcinoma *in situ.* (×100 and ×200)

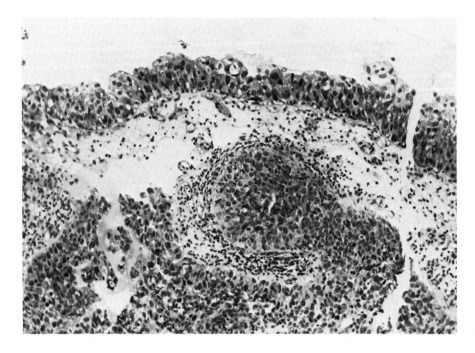

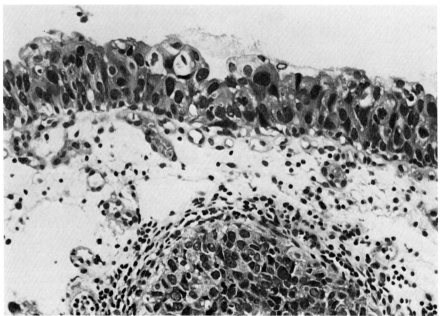

FIGS. 8.11, 8.12.   Carcinoma *in situ* overlying invasive carcinoma. (×40 and ×100)

Chapter 9

Invasive Carcinoma

Aschner (1) in 1931 classified bladder carcinomas as to whether they did or did not invade the underlying tissue. On the basis of a follow-up of 3 years or longer, Aschner found that in lesions without invasion 54% were arrested whereas in carcinomas with invasion 18% were arrested. Aschner concluded that the presence or absence of infiltration represented a reliable guide to the gravity of carcinoma of the bladder.

Jewett and Strong (2) in a classic paper in 1946 demonstrated that there was a relationship between the depth of bladder wall infiltration and the potential curability of bladder carcinoma. Jewett and Strong grouped bladder carcinomas in three stages. The first group (Stage A) included those in which the tumor was confined to the submucosa. The second group (Stage B) consisted of those in which infiltration had extended into the muscularis but not through it. The third group (Stage C) comprised those in which carcinoma had invaded beyond the muscle. From autopsy material Jewett and Strong hypothesized that 100% of patients with superficial tumors confined to the submucosa, 80% of patients whose tumors were confined to the muscularis, and only 26% of patients whose tumors had penetrated into the perivesical fat are potentially curable when first seen.

McDonald and Thompson (3) at the Mayo Clinic immediately provided support for Jewett's concept that the stage of the tumor correlated with survival. McDonald and Thompson studied 272 bladder carcinomas and found that 38.3% of Stage A lesions, 29.6% of Stage B lesions, and 5.2% of Stage C lesions survived 5 years.

Jewett later suggested the segregation of Stage B lesions into superficial (Stage B_1) and deep (Stage B_2) stating that "regardless of histological patterns and degree of malignancy, tumors which have infiltrated less than half-way through the musculature usually are still confined to the bladder wall and tumors which have infiltrated more deeply usually have spread beyond" (4). Marshall (5) in 1952 slightly modified Jewett's staging scheme (Table 1). Prout in 1977 introduced a TNM system of staging (see Table 1) (6).

Marshall demonstrated that there was a strong correlation between the grade and the stage. When the grade of the tumor was low, the stage was also likely to be low. Conversely, when the grade of the tumor was high the stage was also likely to be high. In a study of 107 patients with bladder carcinoma, Marshall found deviations from this association in only seven cases (5).

Although staging became accepted as a valuable aid in determining appropriate therapy for bladder carcinoma, limitations to the value of staging were soon recognized. Marshall reported understaging in 34% of patients who were clinically

TABLE 1.

Jewett-Strong-Marshall	American Joint Committee
O—Epithelial	TIS, Ta (papillary carcinoma confined to mucosa)
A—Lamina propria	T_1
B_1—Superficial muscle	T_2
B_2—Deep muscle	T_3a
C—Perivesical fat	T_3b
D_1—Adjacent organs	T_4—Adjacent organs
Lymph nodes	
	N+ —Pelvic lymph nodes metastases
	M+ —Metastatic lesions other than nodes. Where used, "p" indicates pathological stage specifically

Stage A or B_1. A few of these patients actually had pelvic spread of tumor. Patients who were clinically Stage B_2 or C were found to have a 50% chance of understaging and a 13% chance of overstaging. Consequently, in Stages B_2 and C only 37% of cases were accurately staged clinically (5).

In a study of 90 cases treated by radical surgery shortly after the evaluation of a biopsy specimen, Bergkvist et al. (7) found that in no less than 67 of the 90 cases (75%), the biopsy yielded inaccurate information as to the depth of growth of the tumor. This was partly due to the inadequacy of the biopsy material and partly due to a definite understatement of the depth of growth of the biopsy specimens. The inaccuracy of evaluating the depth of growth based on biopsy specimens increased with the degree of malignancy of the tumor.

Although it is widely held that the evaluation of invasion is the single most important prognostic finding that can be made by the pathologist, it is also recognized that accurately determining the depth of invasion has proved to be difficult. Consequently, many investigators argue that the depth of invasion is far less significant than the presence of invasion. These investigators argue that attempts to assess depth of penetration may result in error and confusion over management. It appears that the most valuable information the pathologist can contribute to the management of the patient is an accurate assessment of the presence or absence of invasion. Difficulties can arise in the estimation of possible invasion of superficial connective tissue, but this question can usually be resolved by studying histological sections from deeper levels of the paraffin block or sections from re-embedded tissue specimens.

In addition to the presence of invasion, it has long been known that lymphatic or vascular invasion affects the accuracy of staging and prognosis. McDonald and Thompson (3) noted lymphatic and venous invasion in 30% of 274 bladder specimens. Lymphatic invasion was three times as great as venous invasion, but they frequently coexisted. Baker (8) found that 20 to 30% of B_1 lesions, 25 to 40% of Stage B_2 lesions, and most Stage C lesions show lymphatic or venous dissemination. Baker did not observe lymphatic spread in Stage A cancers although this has been reported in subsequent studies. Jewett (9) has demonstrated that lymphatic invasion is a dire prognostic event even when the tumor is found only in the lamina propria. Bell et al. (10) have demonstrated poor survival rates in patients with vascular invasion.

HISTOLOGY OF INVASIVE BLADDER CARCINOMA

Invasive bladder carcinomas usually contain several histological patterns that hinder attempts to classify concisely the histological type. The Tumor Registry Committee of the American Urological Association studied 1,224 bladder carcinomas in 1936 and concluded that "it is impracticable to attempt the segregation of bladder tumors into definite groups corresponding to their cell type" (11).

Jewett (12) in 1946 studied 95 autopsy cases in an attempt to classify the tumors into histological groups. Jewett stated:

We immediately encountered difficulties. There were 95 cases in which fairly large blocks, or multiple pieces, had been taken from the primary tumor. Only 48 (51%) of these consisted of a homogeneous histologic pattern with practically the same degree of cellular differentiation throughout the available sections. Twenty-six (27%) consisted of a homogeneous pattern, but showed variation in the degree of differentiation in different parts of the same tumor. There were 21 cases (22%) in which the tumor was papillary in some places and epidermoid in other places, and in some of the cases there was also a considerable variation in the degree of cellular differentiation.

Jewett concluded that "accurate classification of large infiltrating carcinoma of the bladder on the basis of cellular differentiation alone is impossible."

Study after study has confirmed the impressions of the Tumor Registry Committee of the American Urological Association and Jewett. Most invasive bladder carcinomas, if thoroughly sectioned and examined, show foci of transitional, squamous, and glandular differentiation. However, bladder carcinomas are usually divided into the three following major groups.

Transitional Cell Carcinoma

Transitional cell carcinoma (Figs. 9.1–9.8) is by far the most common type of invasive bladder carcinoma. Depending on the histological criteria of the pathologist and the geographical location of the population under study, over 90% of invasive bladder carcinoma will be primarily transitional cell carcinoma.

It has been shown that approximately 20 to 30% of transitional cell carcinomas of the bladder will show evidence of mucin production, and a similar, but not necessarily identical, percentage will show some form of adenomatous metaplasia or glandular configuration. These areas of mucin production and adenomatous metaplasia do not affect the grading of any particular tumor and are seen with equal frequency in low, intermediate, and high grade tumors. These tumors behave biologically as transitional cell carcinomas and should be treated as such (13).

Focal areas of squamous differentiation are frequently found in transitional cell carcinomas. In a study of 2,681 bladder carcinomas, areas of squamous differentiation were seen in about 60% of cases (14). Whether or not the areas of squamous differentiation improve or worsen prognosis has not been determined with certainty.

However, unless the tumors are primarily composed of squamous carcinoma, it is customary to classify these tumors as transitional cell carcinoma.

Squamous Carcinoma

Areas of focal squamous differentiation (Figs. 9.9–9.16) have been found in up to 60% of bladder tumors in some series. However, most of these lesions are predominantly transitional in appearance and behavior, although more frequently they are high grade neoplasms. Pure squamous carcinomas of the bladder comprise 3 to 5% of all bladder tumors (15,16).

The histological criteria necessary for a diagnosis of squamous carcinoma are: (a) the specimen should be overwhelmingly comprised of squamous carcinoma and (b) there should be keratin formation and/or intracellular bridges.

Squamous carcinomas are usually divided into four grades. Grade 1 carcinomas consist of sheets of cells with abundant, homogeneous eosinophilic cytoplasm, intracellular bridges, and round-to-oval nuclei. Whorls of laminated superficial cells may form keratin pearls. Grades 2 and 3 squamous carcinomas show a less orderly maturation with large dark nuclei with prominent nucleoli. Mitoses may be numerous and bizarre. Grade 4 squamous carcinomas show anaplastic cells that may only focally be identifiable as squamous in origin.

There appear to be several distinct differences in the natural history of pure squamous carcinoma and that of typical transitional cell carcinoma of the bladder. These are:

1. A male-to-female ratio of 1:1 or 2:1 rather than the 3:1 or 4:1 (14–17) ratio in transitional cell carcinoma.

2. Squamous carcinomas are more likely to present with symptoms suggestive of advanced disease.

3. Squamous carcinomas have a worse prognosis. Most series show that 60% to 70% die within 1 year of diagnosis despite therapy (15,16).

Adenocarcinoma

Adenocarcinomas (Figs. 9.17–9.24) primary to the bladder account for approximately 1% of epithelial bladder neoplasms. Metastatic adenocarcinomas and prostatic adenocarcinomas infiltrating the bladder are not infrequently confused with primary bladder adenocarcinoma. Primary bladder adenocarcinomas arise from three major sources: (a) vesical adenocarcinoma arising from altered urothelium such as cystitis cystica or cystitis glandularis; (b) urachal adenocarcinoma; and (c) adenocarcinoma arising in an exstrophic bladder.

Vesical Adenocarcinoma

Vesical adenocarcinomas arise from the bladder urothelium. They may occur in any site of the bladder but are most frequent on the base and ureteric areas. There have been occasional well-documented cases of a gradual transition, over many years, from cystitis glandularis to adenocarcinoma. However, since this occurrence is extremely rare the finding of cystitis glandularis should not be interpreted as placing the patient at increased risk of developing adenocarcinoma. Many cases of adenocarcinoma have cystitis cystica, cystitis glandularis, or Brunn's nests in the surrounding urothelium. This finding in itself is not sufficient to document the origin of adenocarcinoma from these lesions.

The prognosis of vesical adenocarcinoma appears to be similar to that of invasive transitional cell carcinoma of similar stage. Thomas et al. (18) followed 28 patients with vesical adenocarcinoma and found that 16 died within 2 years. Thomas et al. did not find a correlation between the degree of histological differentiation and survival.

Symptoms of vesical adenocarcinoma do not differ from other types of bladder tumors. The most common presenting sign is hematuria. Mucus in the urine is rare but may occur in any type of adenocarcinoma of the bladder.

Urachal Adenocarcinoma

Urachal adenocarcinomas account for almost one-half of all adenocarcinomas primary to the bladder. The other half of adenocarcinomas primary to the bladder are usually vesical in origin. Urachal adenocarcinomas generally arise in the dome of the bladder but may occasionally occur in the anterior wall, usually close to the midline. The histology of urachal adenocarcinomas include all grades of differentiation including papillary adenocarcinoma to signet ring carcinoma.

Diagnostic criteria to confirm an adenocarcinoma of urachal origin are:

1. Tumor at the dome or anterior wall of bladder.
2. Intramural or suprapubic mass.
3. Normal mucosa adjacent to or over the tumor.
4. No evidence of primary tumor elsewhere.

Vesical adenocarcinomas usually occur after the fifth decade of life whereas adenocarcinomas of urachal origin are more likely to occur at a younger age. Urachal adenocarcinomas are asymptomatic until they invade the bladder or achieve a size that can be palpated. Thomas et al. (18) followed 28 patients with vesical adenocarcinomas and found that 16 died within 2 years whereas only 5 of 24 urachal adenocarcinomas died during a similar follow-up period. However, Mostofi et al. reported that urachal adenocarcinomas gave very poor prognoses, probably because of incomplete removal of tumor extension (19).

Exstrophy

Adenocarcinoma arising in an exstrophied bladder occurs much less frequently than adenocarcinoma of vesical or urachal origin. However, adenocarcinoma is the most common type of carcinoma arising in exstrophied bladders. Goyanna et al. (20) found 29 cases of carcinoma in exstrophied bladders reported in the literature. Twenty-four of these were adenocarcinoma, two were squamous carcinoma, and three were unidentified carcinoma. Abelhouse (21) reviewed 27 cases of carcinoma in exstrophied bladders and found that 21 were adenocarcinomas, three were squamous carcinoma, and three were carcinoma of undetermined origin.

Adenocarcinomas arising in exstrophied bladders occur at a slightly younger age than adenocarcinomas in normal bladders. This is probably in part a reflection of the shorter life expectancy of patients with exstrophy of the bladder. Adenocarcinomas in exstrophied bladders occur in the third decade of life or later. The peak incidence is in the fifth decade of life.

DIRECT EXTENSION AND METASTATIC BLADDER CARCINOMA

The overall incidence of lymph node metastases in patients undergoing radical cystectomy for bladder carcinoma at the Memorial Sloan Kettering Cancer Center has varied around 20%. The occurrence of lymph node metastases has correlated with the stage of the tumor. Tumors invading the lamina propria (Stage A) had a 5% incidence of lymph node metastases, tumors invading the superficial muscle (Stage B_1) had a 13% incidence of lymph node metastases, tumors invading the deep muscle (Stage B_2) had an 18% incidence of lymph node metastases, and tumors extending beyond the deep muscle (Stages C and D) had a 44% incidence of lymph node metastases. Patients with muscle invasion without demonstrable lymph node metastases are at an approximately 50% risk of developing evidence of disseminated bladder carcinoma (22).

Jewett (2) studied 52 autopsy cases of metastatic bladder carcinoma and found that regional lymph nodes were the site of metastases in 33 instances, the liver in 26, the lungs in 18, and the vertebral column, including the sacrum and pelvis, in 11. Other tissues were involved 20 times, but in only 7.7% of the cases without involvement of lymph nodes, liver, lungs, or bone. In 36.5% of the cases in which metastases were found, the regional lymph nodes were not involved. Melicow (23), in an autopsy study of 125 consecutive cases of bladder tumors, found visceral metastases in 106 cases. The liver, lungs, adrenals, and kidneys were most commonly involved. Less commonly involved were the heart, diaphragm, gall bladder, pancreas, colon, and small intestine. The retroperitoneum was at times massively involved with local extension of the tumor.

The histological characteristics of the metastatic bladder carcinoma do not consistently mirror the histological characteristics of the primary tumor. Jewett studied 14 cases of metastatic bladder carcinoma in which the primary tumor showed a homogeneous histological pattern and 25 cases in which the primary tumor was known not to be homogeneous. In only 8 of the 14 supposedly homogeneous cases, the histology of the metastases were similar to the primary tumor. Of the 25 cases of nonhomogeneous tumors that had metastasized, the histology of the metastases were similar to the primary tumor in only 11 cases (12).

The presence of lymph node metastases has been an ominous prognostic feature. In one study of 11 patients treated by total cystectomy in whom lymph node metastases were present, there were no 5-year survivors (24). Other studies have shown 10 to 40% 5-year survivals of patients with metastases to lymph nodes (25,26,27). The more favorable survivals were usually possible after meticulous pelvic node dissection.

REFERENCES

1. Aschner, P. W. (1931): Clinical application of bladder tumor pathology. *Surg. Gynecol. Obstet.*, 52:979–1000.
2. Jewett, H. J., and Strong, G. H. (1946): Infiltrating carcinoma of the bladder: relationship of depth of penetration of the bladder wall to incidence of local extension and metastases. *J. Urol.*, 55:366–372.
3. McDonald, J. R., and Thompson, G. T. (1948): Carcinoma of the urinary bladder: a pathologic study with special reference to invasiveness and vascular invasion. *J. Urol.*, 60:435–445.
4. Jewett, H. J. (1952): Carcinoma of the bladder: influence of depth of infiltration on the 5-year results following extirpation of the primary growth. *J. Urol.*, 67:672–680.
5. Marshall, V. F. (1952): The relation of the pre-operative estimate to the pathologic demonstration of the extent of vesical neoplasms. *J. Urol.*, 68:714–723.
6. Prout, G. R. (1977): Bladder carcinoma and a TNM system of classification. *J. Urol.*, 117:583–590.
7. Bergkvist, A., Ljungqvist, A., and Moberger, G. (1965): Classification of bladder tumors based on cellular pattern: preliminary report of a clinicopathological study of 300 cases with a minimum follow-up of 8 years. *Acta Chir. Scand.*, 130:371–378.
8. Baker, R. (1968): The accuracy of clinical vs. surgical staging. *JAMA*, 206:1770–1773.
9. Jewett, H. J., King, L. R., and Shelley, W. M. (1964): A study of 365 cases of infiltrating bladder cancer. *J. Urol.*, 92:668–678.
10. Bell, J. T., Berney, S. W., and Friedell, G. F. (1971): Blood vessel invasion in human bladder cancer. *J. Urol.*, 105:675–678.
11. Tumor Registry Committee (1936): Grading of epithelial tumors of the urinary bladder: a study of the cell types and the method of grading of the cases in the carcinoma registry of the American Urological Association. *J. Urol.*, 36:651–668.
12. Jewett, H. J., and Blackman, S. S. (1946): Infiltrating carcinoma of the bladder: histologic pattern and degree of cellular differentiation in 97 autopsy cases. *J. Urol.*, 56:200–210.
13. Ward, A. M. (1971): Glandular metaplasia and mucin production in transitional cell carcinoma of bladder. *J. Clin. Pathol.*, 24:481.
14. Sarma, K. P. (1970): Squamous cell carcinoma of the bladder. *Int. Surg.*, 53:313–319.
15. Bessette, P. L., Abell, M. R., and Herwig, K. R. (1974): A clinicopathological study of squamous cell carcinoma of the bladder. *J. Urol.*, 112:66–67.
16. Newman, D. M., Brown, J. R., Jay, A. C., and Pontius, E. E. (1968): Squamous cell carcinoma of the bladder. *J. Urol.*, 100:470–473.
17. Miller, A., Mitchell, J. P., and Brown, N. J. (1969): The Bristol bladder tumour registry. *Br. J. Urol. (suppl)*, 41:1–64.
18. Thomas, D. G., Ward, A. M., and Williams, J. L. (1971): A study of 52 cases of adenocarcinoma of the bladder. *Br. J. Urol.*, 43:4–15.
19. Mostofi, F. K., Thomson, R. V., and Dean, A. L. (1955): Mucous adenocarcinoma of the bladder. *Cancer*, 8:741–758.
20. Goyanna, R., Emmett, J. L., McDonald, R. (1951): Exstrophy of the bladder complicated by adenocarcinoma. *J. Urol.*, 65:391–400.
21. Abeshouse, B. S.: Exstrophy of the bladder complicated by adenocarcinoma of the bladder and renal calculi. *J. Urol.*, 49:259–289.
22. Whitmore, W. F., Jr. (1982): Editorial comment. *J. Urol.*, 128:36.
23. Melicow, M. M. (1974): Tumors of the bladder: a multifaceted problem. *J. Urol.*, 112:467–478.
24. Cordonnier, J. J. (1968): Cystectomy for carcinoma of the bladder. *J. Urol.*, 99:172–173.
25. Dretler, S. P., Ragsdale, B. D., and Leadbetter, W. F. (1973): The value of pelvic lymphadenectomy in the surgical treatment of bladder cancer. *J. Urol.*, 109:414–416.
26. Whitmore, W. F., Jr., and Marshall, V. F. (1962): Radical total cystectomy for cancer of the bladder: 230 consecutive cases five years later. *J. Urol.*, 87:853–868.
27. Skinner, D. G. (1982): Management of invasive bladder carcinoma: a meticulous pelvic node dissection can make a difference. *J. Urol.*, 128:34–36.

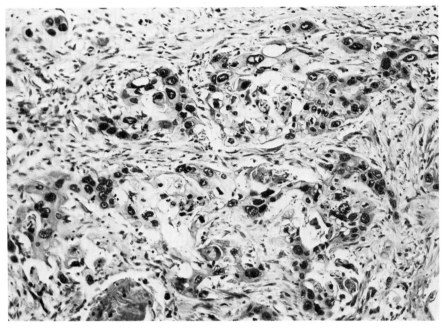

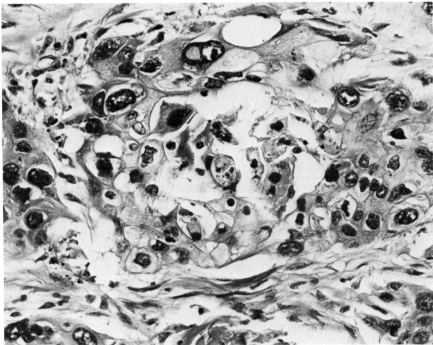

FIGS. 9.1, 9.2. Invasive transitional cell carcinoma. ($\times 100$ and $\times 200$)

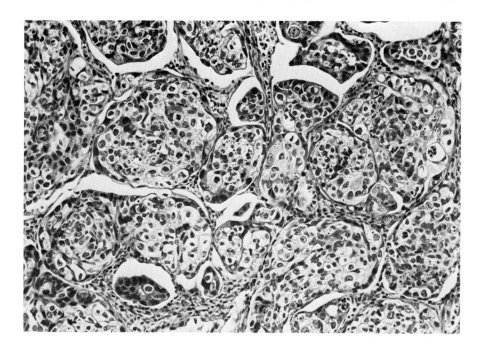

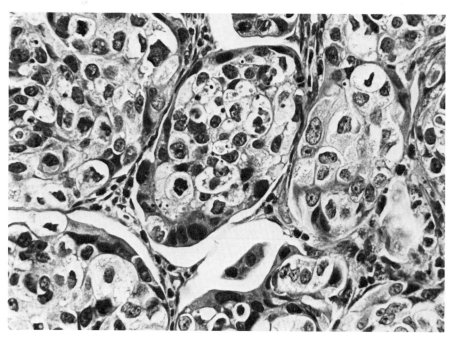

FIGS. 9.3, 9.4. Invasive transitional cell carcinoma. (×100 and ×200)

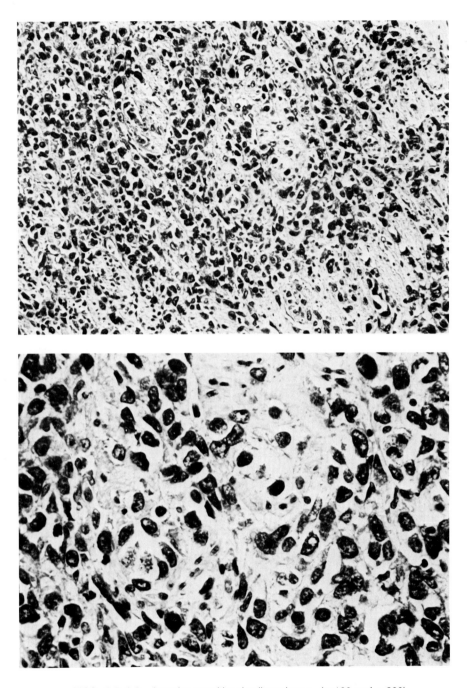

FIGS. 9.5, 9.6.   Invasive transitional cell carcinoma. (×100 and ×200)

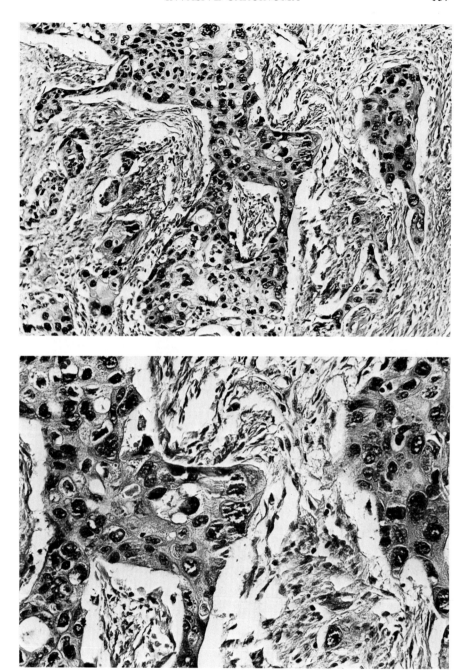

FIGS. 9.7, 9.8. Invasive transitional cell carcinoma. (×100 and ×200)

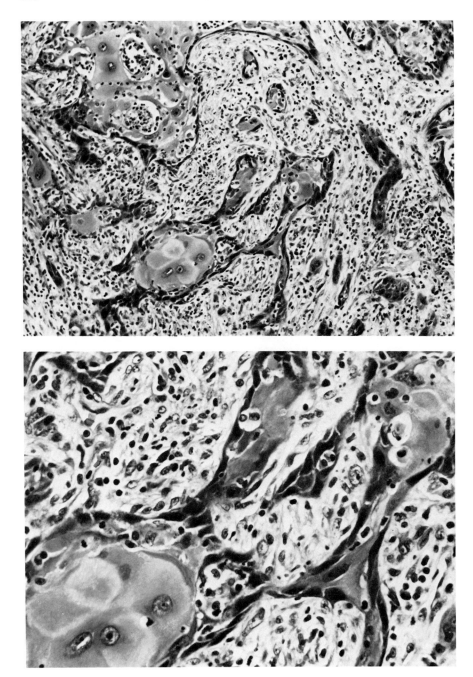

FIGS. 9.9, 9.10. Squamous carcinoma. ($\times$ 100 and $\times$ 200)

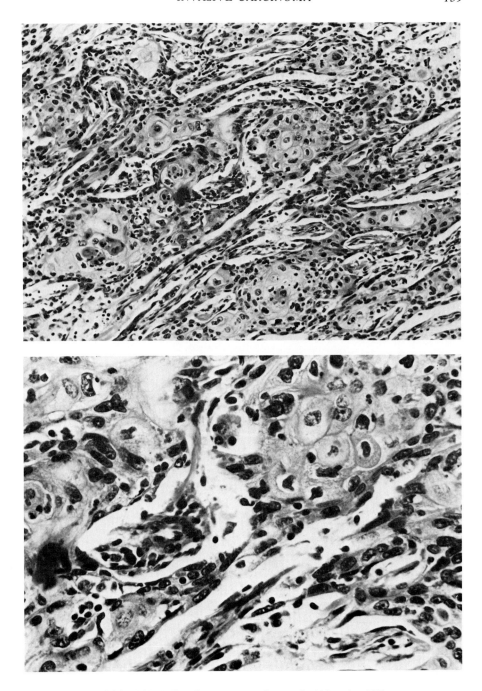

FIGS. 9.11, 9.12. Squamous carcinoma. ($\times$100 and $\times$200)

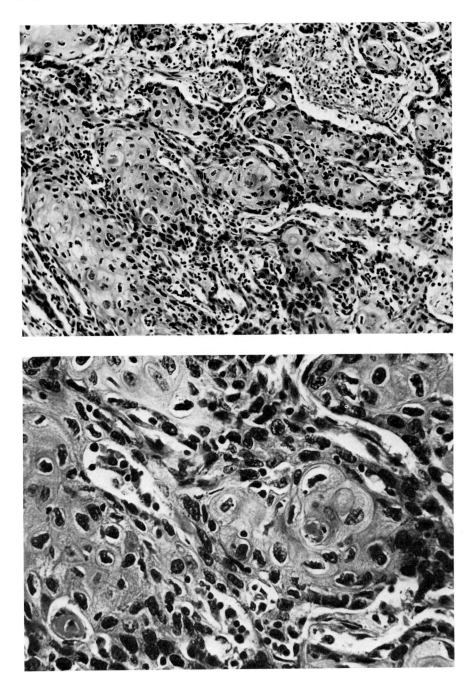

FIGS. 9.13, 9.14.   Squamous carcinoma. ($\times$100 and $\times$200)

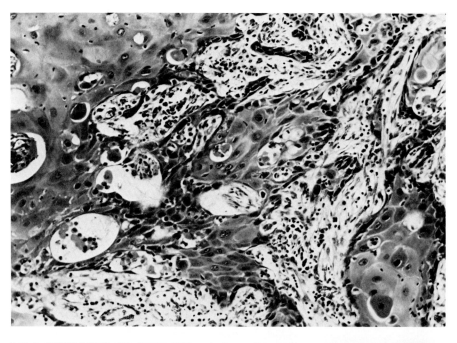

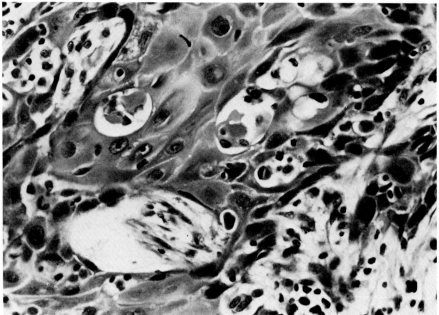

FIGS. 9.15, 9.16. Squamous carcinoma. (×100 and ×200)

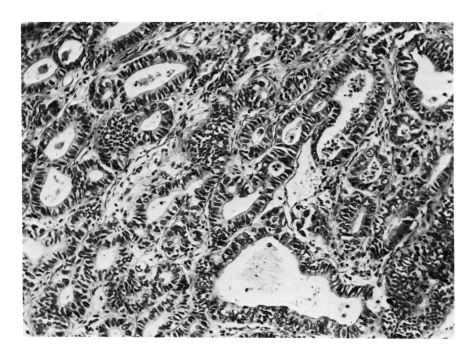

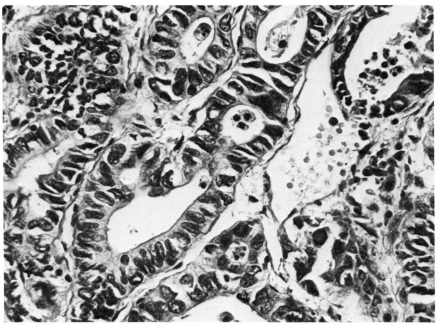

FIGS. 9.17, 9.18.   Adenocarcinoma. ($\times$100 and $\times$200)

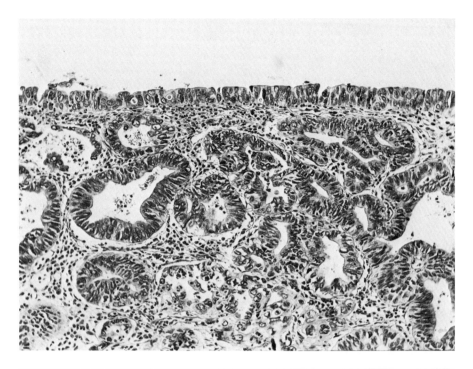

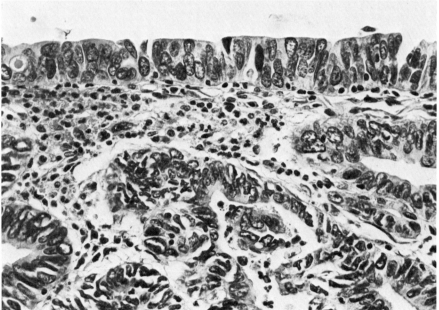

FIGS. 9.19, 9.20. Adenocarcinoma. ($\times 100$ and $\times 200$)

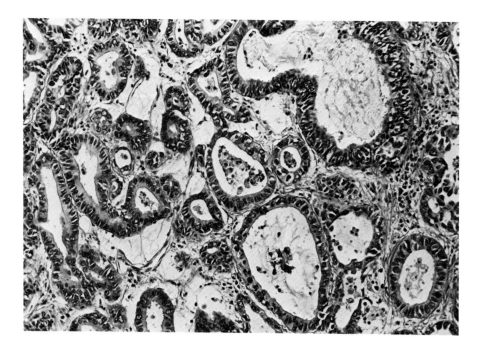

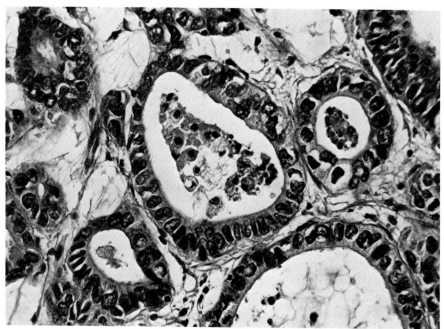

FIGS. 9.21, 9.22. Adenocarcinoma. ($\times$100 and $\times$200)

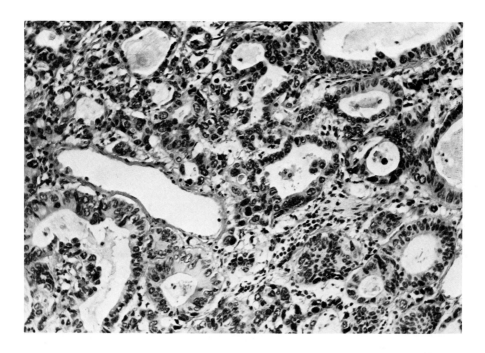

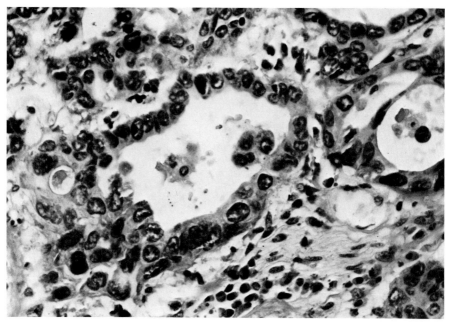

FIGS. 9.23, 9.24. Adenocarcinoma. (×100 and ×200)

Chapter 10

Cytology

The first study of exfoliated cancer cells from bladder carcinoma is credited to Sanders (1) who in 1865 found malignant cells in urine from a patient with extensive bladder carcinoma. Ferguson (2) in 1892 suggested that microscopic examination of urine sediment was the best method besides cystoscopy for diagnosing tumors of the bladder. In 1925 Parameter (3) presented the first standard approach to the examination of urine as an aid in the diagnosis of tumors of the genitourinary tract. However, it was not until Papanicolaou (4) in 1945 published a series of 83 cases of urine cytology that this field began to be thoroughly investigated. In Papanicolaou's original paper, 27 cases were reported as positive for neoplasm on the basis of smear without any knowledge of the clinical findings. In 24 of these (89%), the cytology diagnosis was confirmed either by biopsy (21 cases) or by clinical findings (3 cases).

Cytological examination of the urinary sediment began to be used as a routine method of cancer detection in the 1950s by Crabbe (5) on British dyestuff workers and Koss and Melamed (6) on industrial workers exposed to para-aminodiphenyl. In those groups with a high expected incidence of bladder carcinoma, cytological studies helped curtail the frequency of cystoscopies and led to a number of diagnoses of cancer months or years before the disease could be identified cystoscopically.

NORMAL URINARY SEDIMENT

Urothelial cells in normal urinary sediment (Figs. 10.1, 10.2) are few in number. The finding of a clean background, the absence of cell detritus, and the presence of a few well-recognizable cells of the various layers should suffice for a benign cytological report. In the event of a negative cytological report, a repeat examination is warranted in proportion to the degree of clinical suspicion.

The normal cells in urine arise mostly from the transitional epithelium of the urinary tract and vary greatly in size, shape, and appearance. It is this variation in the morphology of exfoliated transitional cells that is responsible for some of the difficulty in the interpretation of urinary sediment. The superficial layer of the bladder normally sheds multinucleated cells. Since multinucleated tumor cells are rarely seen in urine sediment, the finding of multinucleated cells in urine is usually a sign of benignity. The intermediate layers of the urothelium exfoliate elongated cells whereas the deeper layers exfoliate smaller cells with a darker nucleus. These smaller cells are characterized by relatively large nuclei with dense nuclear membranes and only a few scattered, fine chromatin clumps, with otherwise empty-appearing nuclei. In about 50% of all adult females, the trigone of the bladder

146

contains areas of mature squamous epithelium similar to that found in the vagina. Squamous cells in the urinary sediment can arise either from these areas of squamous metaplasia or from superficial squamous cells of the urethra. It is only in disease of the urinary tract that blood, pus, or debris are present in any quantity.

INFLAMMATION

In the presence of inflammation or irritative phenomena, there is usually an increased exfoliation of cells of transitional epithelial origin. These cells are frequently of bizarre shapes, often binucleated or multinucleated, and sometimes substantially enlarged. The nuclei vary in size, may display slight hyperchromasia, losing their normal "empty" appearance, and may occasionally contain small nucleoli. The nuclear-cytoplasmic ratio is not significantly altered. Cytoplasmic vacuolization, sometimes with engulfed leukocytes may occur. Occasionally intracytoplasmic globular, irregular, or fragmented eosinophilic inclusions occur. These inclusions are more commonly seen in degenerating cells and have no diagnostic significance.

A rare disease of the urinary bladder, malakoplakia, may sometimes be diagnosed in the urinary sediment. Histiocytes with large, sometimes calcified, cytoplasmic inclusions (Michaelis-Gutman bodies) may be observed in the sediment. Other benign abnormalities include herpetic cystitis, cytomegalic inclusion disease, and human polyoma virus.

RADIATION CHANGES

An important source of diagnostic error is radiotherapy. Radiotherapy to the bladder or to adjacent organs such as the uterus may cause abnormalities characterized by marked but variable cell enlargement, usually including both the nucleus and the cytoplasm. The nucleus is generally more affected than the cytoplasm, and the nuclear changes appear to precede cytoplasmic abnormalities. The enlarged nucleus is often eccentric, slightly irregular in outline, and nearly always markedly hyperchromatic. The chromatin granules are at times coarse, but their distribution is fairly even. Chromatin centers or nucleoli are often present. The nucleoli may be large and distorted with irregular and sharp edges.

Among cytologists there is agreement that great caution should be exercised when persistence or recurrence of bladder carcinoma after irradiation is suspected. Cowen (7) has stated that "on review of the literature, we feel that it is impossible to state with any degree of certainty whether any atypical or bizarre cells seen in urine indicate a neoplastic origin, or whether they are due to irradiation of non-neoplastic epithelial cells." L. G. Koss has pointed out that "on occasion the nuclei of irradiated benign cells will display some hyperchromatia that may render the differential diagnosis difficult. When material is sent for cytologic analysis, any previous radiotherapy should clearly be indicated on the request slip" (8).

CHEMOTHERAPY

A variety of chemotherapy agents and their effects on urine sediment have been studied. The urine sediment from patients receiving chemotherapy may contain abnormal cells that cannot be readily distinguished from those of cancer. These abnormal cells are characterized by nuclear hyperchromasia, nuclear enlargement, and abnormal giant cells. The cytoplasm commonly shows marked vacuolization and occasional infiltration by polymorphonuclear leukocytes. Cytoplasmic smudging with long tails may be present, but this may represent mechanical trauma during preparation of the smear. The cellular background may contain numerous erythrocytes, cell debris, and leukocytes.

DECOY CELLS

Papanicolaou recognized the presence of certain atypical cells in some urinary sediment, and because of their shape he named them "comet" cells (9). L. G. Koss and Ricci (8) named the same cells "decoy" cells. These cells are very commonly found in voided urine smears and have many characteristics of malignancy. They are found in both male and female urine from healthy patients as well as in urine containing malignant cells. They consist of round or oval nuclei with a coarse chromatin network. The chromatin can be clumped to appear completely hyperchromatic. There may be a slight tag of cytoplasm attached to the nucleus or this may be completely absent. Occasionally, the cells may be binucleate and vary in size. These "decoy" cells may be few in number or be fairly numerous with 30 to 40 per smear.

The origin of these cells has not been entirely established. They appear to be transitional epithelial cells that are either undergoing degeneration or cells infected with human polyoma virus (HPV).

SEMINAL VESICLES

Cells derived from the epithelial lining of the seminal vesicles or their ducts are ordinarily found in urine specimens after prostatic massage or ejaculation. These cells are often associated with numerous spermatozoa. The cells have a very densely staining homogeneous nuclei that are usually smoothly outlined and eccentrically located. The cells often appear to be degenerating. Some contain a yellow lipochrome pigment within the cytoplasm. Occasionally, the cells can be enlarged and extremely bizarre. If these cells do not contain lipochrome pigment, correct identification can be difficult. Clues as to the origin of these cells are the presence of lipochrome pigment and the presence of additional cells from the seminal vesicles.

LITHIASIS AND RETROGRADE CATHERIZATION

Lithiasis of the lower urinary tract and retrograde catherization may result in the desquamation of large clusters of urothelial cells. The cells dislodged by retrograde catherization are often multinucleated whereas the cells from patients with lithiasis may be multinucleated, elongated, and contain occasional mitotic figures. These clusters of cells may have a papillary configuration that may be confused with papillary tumors. One must be aware that specimens taken from patients with lithiasis or patients undergoing retrograde catherization are not fully reliable for evaluating the significance of papillary fronds.

ATYPICAL HYPERPLASIA/DYSPLASIA

There appears to be a continuum from dysplasia, or atypical hyperplasia, to carcinoma *in situ*. Cytological evaluation of dysplasia is difficult because dysplastic lesions exfoliate few cells, and the exfoliated cells may be distorted by the hostile environment of the urine. However, at the Mayo Clinic, of 279 patients with atypical cytology, 158 were eventually shown to have bladder carcinoma (10).

NEOPLASIA

High grade, high stage lesions are more easily diagnosed than low grade, low stage lesions. The low grade, low stage lesions are the source of most false positive diagnoses. As yet, however, we do not always know what a false positive report really means. The Mayo Clinic followed 203 patients with positive urine cytology and negative cystoscopy findings. Cancer was ultimately identified in 190 of the patients (10). Heney et al. reviewed the cases of 267 patients with positive urine cytology and found 18 with negative cystoscopy findings. Follow-up revealed that 11 of these 18 patients subsequently developed overt urothelial carcinoma after an average of 19 months (11).

Positive urine cytology with negative cystoscopy findings should be followed with multiple random biopsies of the urothelium and repeat cytology studies. In the face of continued positive urine cytology with negative histology on multiple samples of bladder urothelium, the possibility of a primary renal, ureteral, urethral, or prostatic malignancy should be considered. Collection of urine for cytology studies directly from each ureter, the acquisition of ureteral biopsy as appropriate, and transurethral resection of the prostate to provide samples of prostatic ducts/urethra for histological study may all help to locate the disease.

Papillomas

If the lining urothelium of a papillary tumor (Figs. 10.3 to 10.8) closely resembles normal urothelium, then it is unlikely that the cells shed will deviate from normal sufficiently to make a definite diagnosis. The only possible indication to the presence of such a growth will be an abnormally large number of relatively normal transitional cells in the smear.

Some studies (12) have suggested that papillomas can be detected cytologically by the presence of (a) papillomatous fronds, (b) cells with elongated cigar-shaped nuclei, and (c) cells with broad cytoplasmic tails ending in bulbous extremities. However, most investigators have found that individual cell changes such as nuclear pleomorphism and/or hyperchromasia are usually absent even in the presence of cystoscopically visible low grade tumor. Because of the absence of cytological abnormalities, most observers have found that in the presence of papillomas, the urinary sediment will contain no diagnostic cells whatsoever. Malignant cells in urine cytology specimens from patients with papillomas most likely arise from other sites of the bladder than from the papilloma, i.e., foci of a higher grade neoplasm elsewhere in the bladder.

Low Grade Papillary Transitional Cell Carcinomas

Low grade papillary carcinomas (Figs. 10.9 to 10.14) may be diagnosed by examination of cells exfoliated in the urine or bladder washings. Cell morphology is somewhat similar to that seen in papillomas, but nuclear atypia and cell irregularity are slightly increased. Chromatin clumping is more obvious, and the cells are slightly more hyperchromatic than in papillomas. The cytoplasm may be normal in amount or slightly decreased in amount. Clusters of cells similar to those found in low grade transitional papillary carcinomas may also be found in patients following retrograde catherization or in patients with lithiasis.

High Grade Papillary Transitional Cell Carcinomas

Higher grade (Grades 2 and 3) papillary transitional cell carcinomas (Figs. 10.15 to 10.28) usually shed abundant carcinoma cells. These cells may be shed singly or in clusters. It is sometimes possible to distinguish Grade 2 lesions from Grade 3 lesions on cytological examination of the urinary sediment. Urothelial tumors, Grade 2, will usually shed malignant cells in small clusters. The individual cells show enlarged nuclei with moderate anaplasia. Elongated columnar cells may be present. Grade 3 tumors usually shed cells singly with a high degree of nuclear pleomorphism. Degenerative changes such as cytoplasmic vacuolization and nuclear pyknosis are often present.

Carcinoma *In Situ*

Carcinoma *in situ* (Figs. 10.29 to 10.34) characteristically sheds malignant cells singly or in small clusters. The tendency to exfoliate easily probably accounts for the sensitivity of cytological techniques in detecting areas of carcinoma *in situ* that are quite small. Most of the cells are about the size of normal bladder epithelial cells or slightly larger. The nuclei are usually slightly enlarged, round-to-oval, although they may be irregular or angular. The nuclei are invariably hyperchromatic with coarse chromatin. The cytoplasm is not greatly reduced in amount or different from that of normal transitional cells. Red blood cells and leukocytes are sparse.

Carcinoma *in situ* can usually be distinguished from invasive carcinoma. Whereas invasive carcinoma usually shows inflammation and necrosis in the urinary sediment, these findings are not prominent in carcinoma *in situ*. In addition, nuclear alterations within the malignant cells of carcinoma *in situ* are less marked than in invasive carcinoma.

Invasive Carcinomas

Invasive carcinomas (Figs. 10.35, 10.36) of the bladder are usually derivatives of transitional epithelium. The invasive cells are characterized by bizarre nuclear and cytoplasmic configuration with marked individual variation. The nuclei are densely hyperchromatic, enlarged, and irregular in outline. Coarse clumping of chromatin and prominent nucleoli are characteristic of these cells. However, the chromatin detail may be obscured if the cells are degenerating. The cytoplasm of invasive transitional cell carcinomas is usually scanty.

Squamous carcinomas of bladder origin have features similar to squamous carcinomas elsewhere. The cells are characterized by abundant cytoplasm and evidence of keratinization. Adenocarcinomas may present as undifferentiated cells with only a faint background of cytoplasm and no cellular border. More commonly, adenocarcinomas will have a suggestion of acinar formation.

REFERENCES

1. Sanders, W. R. (1865): Cancer of the bladder: fragments forming urethral plugs discharged in urine. *Edinburgh Med. J.*, 10:273–274.
2. Ferguson, F. (1892): The diagnosis of tumors of the bladder by microscopical examination. *Proc. N.Y., Path. Soc. Meeting*, April 27, 1892, p. 71–73.
3. Esposti, P. L., and Zajicek, J. (1972): Grading of transitional cell neoplasms of the urinary bladder from smears of bladder washings: a critical review of 326 tumors. *Acta Cytol.*, 16:529–537.
4. Papanicolaou, G. N., and Marshall, V. F. (1945): Urine sediment smears as a diagnostic procedure in cancer of the urinary tract. *Science*, 101:519.
5. Crabbe, J. G. S., Cresdee, W. C., Scott, T. S., and Williams, M. H. C. (1956): The cytological diagnosis of bladder tumours amongst dyestuff workers. *Br. J. Ind. Med.*, 13:270–276.
6. Koss, L. G., Melamed, W. R., Ricci, A., Melick, W. F., and Kelly, R. E. (1965): Carcinogenesis in the human urinary bladder: observation after exposure to para-aminodiphenyl. *N. Engl. J. Med.*, 272:767–770.
7. Cowen, P. N. (1975): False cytodiagnosis of bladder malignancy due to previous radiotherapy. *Br. J. Urol.*, 47:405–412.
8. Koss, L. G. (1968): *Diagnostic Cytology and Its Histopathologic Basis*, 2nd edition, pp. 404–452. J. B. Lippincott, Philadelphia.
9. Papanicolaou, G. N. (1954): The urinary and male genital systems. In: *Atlas of Exfoliative Cytology*. Commonwealth Fund, Harvard University Press, Cambridge, Massachusetts.
10. Utz, D. C., Farrow, G. M., Rife, C. C., Segura, J. W., and Zincke, H. (1980): Carcinoma in situ of the bladder. *Cancer*, 45:1842–1848.
11. Daly, J. J. Carcinoma-in-situ of the urothelium. *Urol. Clin. North Am.* (February 1976), Vol. 3, No. 1:87–105.
12. Allegra, S. R., Broderick, P. A., and Corvese, N. L. (1972): Cytologic and histogenetic observations in well differentiated transitional cell carcinoma of bladder. *J. Urol.*, 107:777–782.

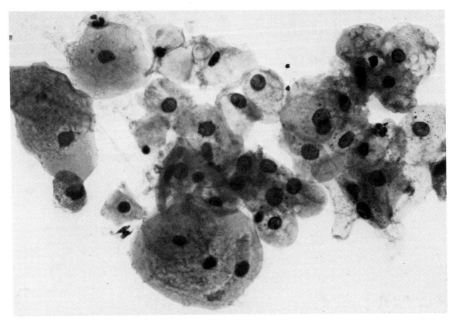

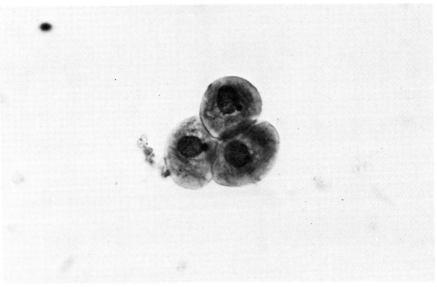

FIGS. 10.1, 10.2. Normal urinary cytology. (×400)

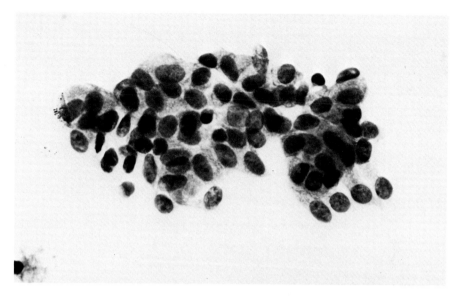

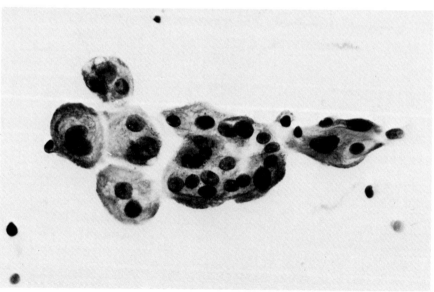

FIGS. 10.3, 10.4. Urinary cytology from patients with papillomas. (×400)

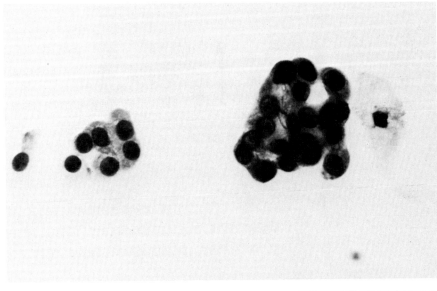

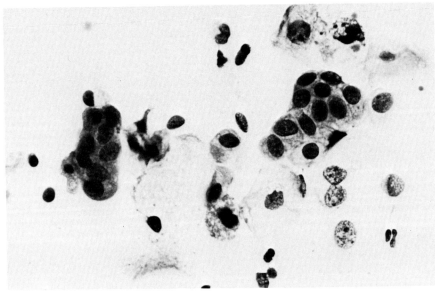

FIGS. 10.5, 10.6. Urinary cytology from patients with papillomas. (×400)

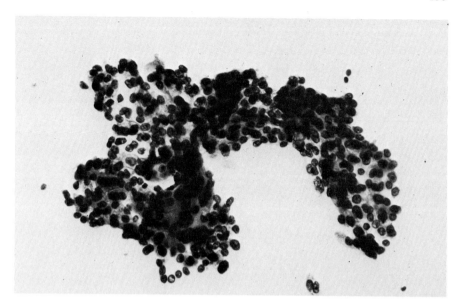

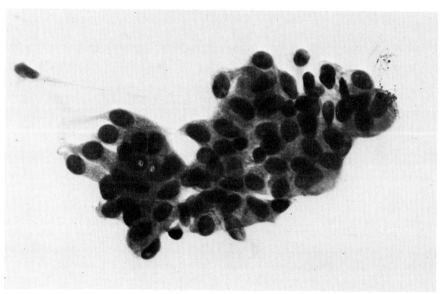

FIGS. 10.7, 10.8. Urinary cytology from patients with papillomas. (×400)

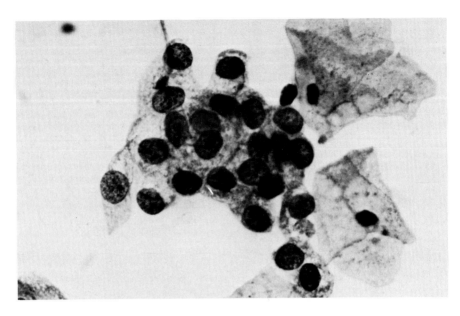

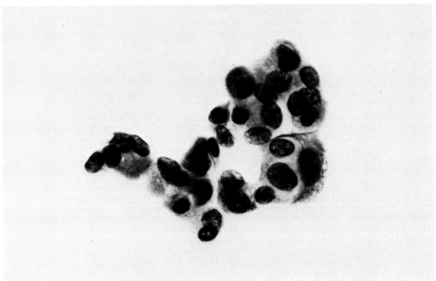

FIGS. 10.9, 10.10. Urinary cytology from patients with Grade 1 papillary tumors. ($\times 400$)

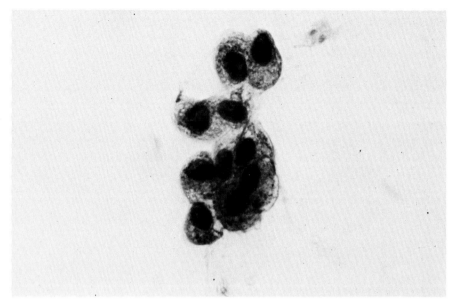

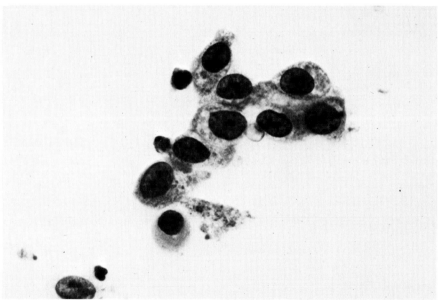

FIGS. 10.11, 10.12. Urinary cytology from patients with Grade 1 papillary tumors. ($\times$400)

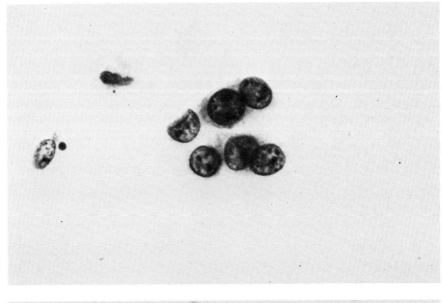

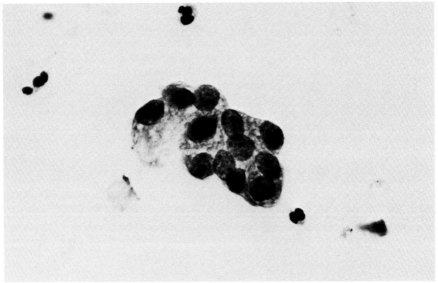

FIGS. 10.13, 10.14. Urinary cytology from patients with Grade 1 papillary tumors. ($\times 400$)

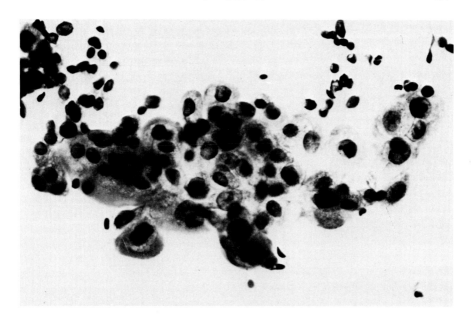

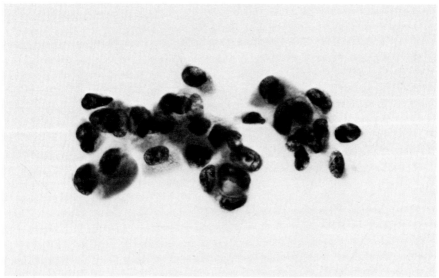

FIGS. 10.15, 10.16. Urinary cytology from patients with Grade 2 papillary tumors. ($\times$ 400)

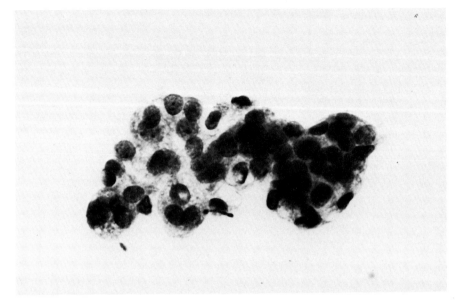

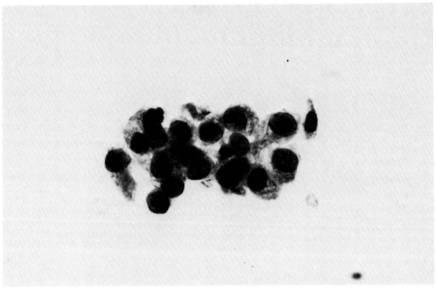

FIGS. 10.17, 10.18.   Urinary cytology from patients with Grade 2 papillary tumors. ($\times$ 400)

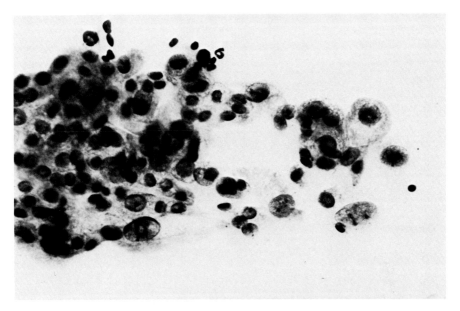

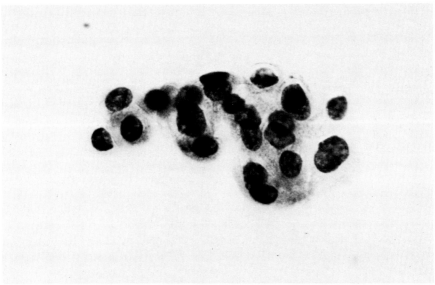

FIGS. 10.19, 10.20. Urinary cytology from patients with Grade 2 papillary tumors. ($\times$400)

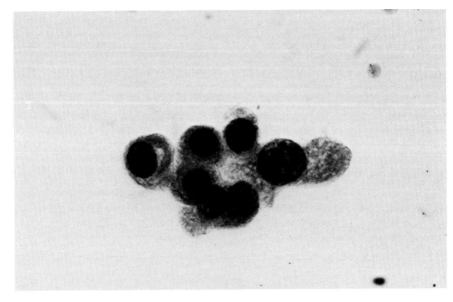

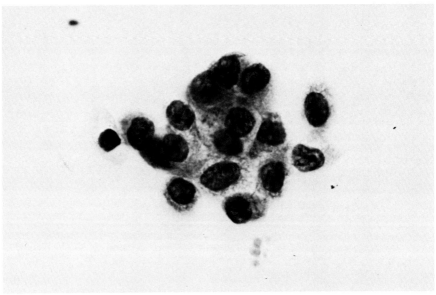

FIGS. 10.21, 10.22. Urinary cytology from patients with Grade 2 papillary tumors. (×400)

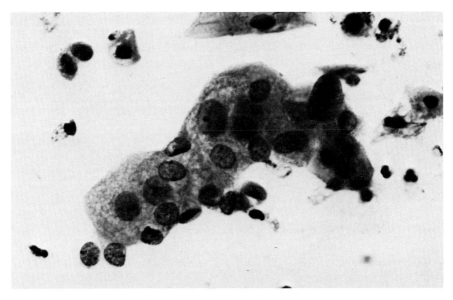

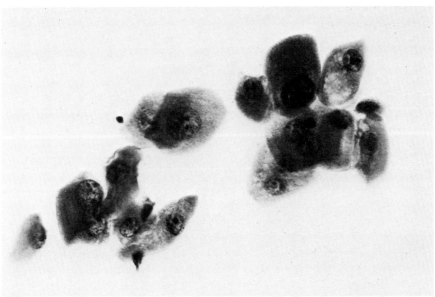

FIGS. 10.23, 10.24. Urinary cytology from patients with Grade 2 papillary tumors. (×400)

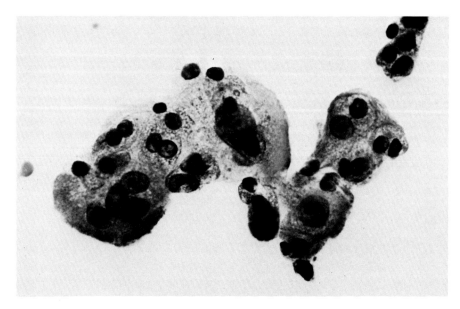

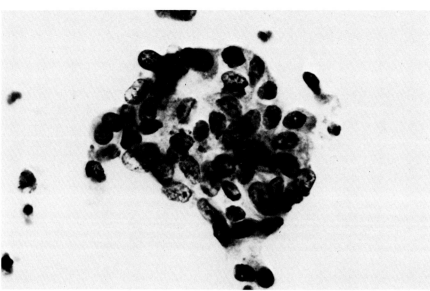

FIGS. 10.25, 10.26. Urinary cytology from patients with Grade 3 papillary tumors. (×400)

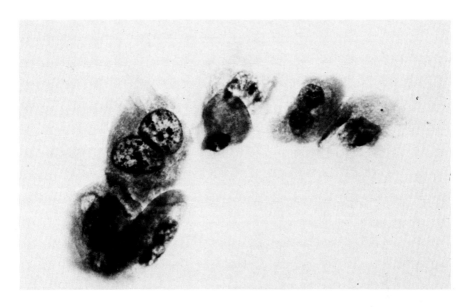

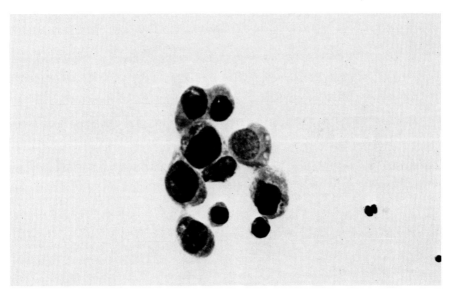

FIGS. 10.27, 10.28. Urinary cytology from patients with Grade 3 papillary tumors. (×400)

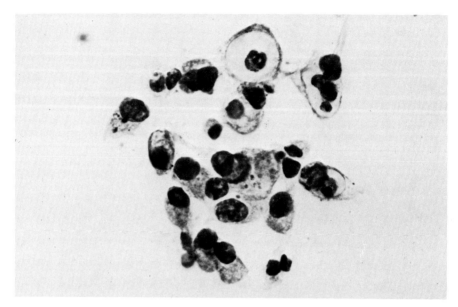

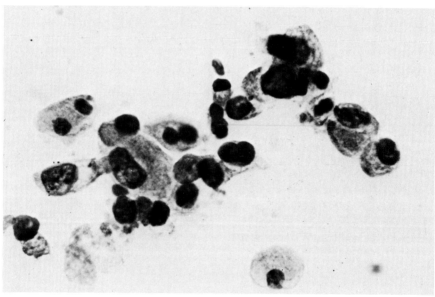

FIGS. 10.29, 10.30. Urinary cytology from patients with carcinoma *in situ*. (×400)

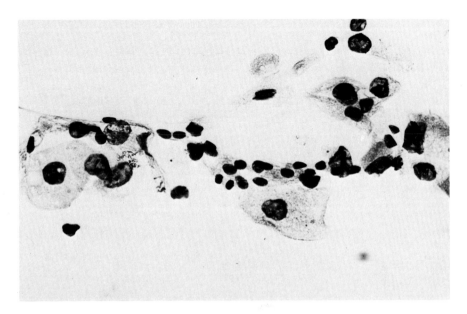

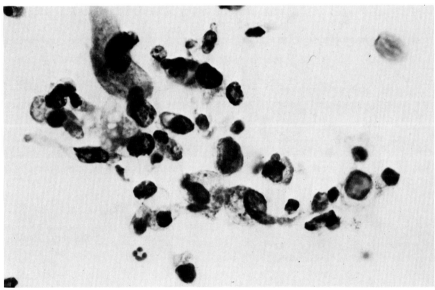

FIGS. 10.31, 10.32. Urinary cytology from patients with carcinoma *in situ*. (×400)

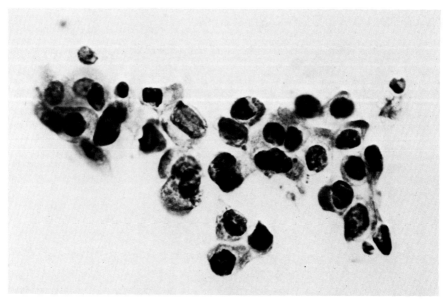

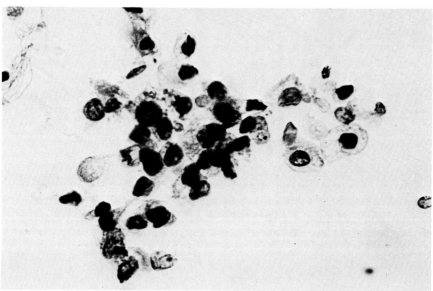

FIGS. 10.33, 10.34. Urinary cytology from patients with carcinoma *in situ*. (×400)

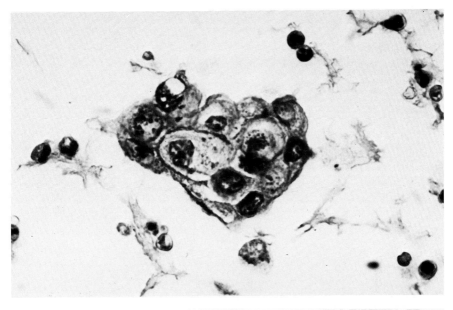

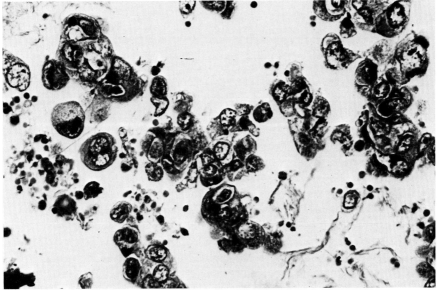

FIGS. 10.35, 10.36. Urinary cytology from patients with invasive bladder carcinoma. (×400)

Chapter 11

Miscellaneous Nonmalignant Bladder Lesions

SQUAMOUS METAPLASIA

Squamous metaplasia (Figs. 11.1 to 11.6) occurs when the normal bladder urothelium is altered to resemble squamous epithelium. Squamous metaplasia is one of the first mucosal alterations occurring in exstrophied bladders. In exstrophied bladders squamous metaplasia is usually extensive and can resemble normal skin. In normally developed bladders focal areas of squamous metaplasia are common. Packham (1) biopsied 50 trigones in women with abacterial recurrent cystitis and found squamous metaplasia in 42 (84%). Koss (2) found squamous metaplasia in 22 of 100 normal bladders during post-mortem studies.

Squamous metaplasia is more common and extensive in women than in men and is most often found at the bladder neck or trigone. Inflammation is not invariably seen associated with squamous metaplasia. However, it is possible that some cases of squamous metaplasia may have been initiated by inflammation and that after the inflammation resolved the squamous metaplasia persisted.

Squamous metaplasia appears to be a normal variant of urothelium in most cases. However, in other cases squamous metaplasia is an adaptive reactive process in which the less resistant urothelium is replaced by more resistant squamous epithelium. Squamous metaplasia may interfere with the normal contracture and dilatation of the bladder. Squamous metaplasia does not appear to be as efficient in maintaining the urine blood barrier as normal urothelium.

Squamous metaplasia has been found in 72% (3) of cases of squamous carcinoma associated with schistosomiasis. However, in this setting, it is not known whether the squamous metaplasia is a forerunner, fellow traveler, or follower of squamous carcinoma. The first case of squamous metaplasia in an otherwise normal bladder progressing to carcinoma was reported by Holley and Mellinger in 1961 (4). A similar case was reported by Kelalis, Emmett, and DeWeerd in 1963 (5), and additional cases were reported by O'Flynn and Mullaney in 1967 (6). Although the association of squamous metaplasia and squamous carcinoma occasionally occurs, there is no convincing evidence that the squamous metaplasia frequently found in women is a premalignant condition.

ENDOMETRIOSIS

The first description of endometriosis of the bladder (Figs. 11.7, 11.8) was by Judd (7) at the Mayo Clinic in 1921. Endometriosis of the bladder represents a small percentage of cases of pelvic endometriosis. Ball and Platt (8) reported 14 cases of bladder involvement in a total of 720 cases with pelvic endometrial implants.

Endometriosis may involve the bladder either as an isolated finding or in association with endometriosis elsewhere. Most cases are localized on the serosal side and asymptomatic. Endometriosis of the bladder may occur in any woman between menarche and menopause. In the majority of cases, it occurs between the ages of 25 and 40 with the greatest number in patients between 30 and 35 (9).

The endometrial lesion is usually single but may be multiple and vary in size from a small discrete plaque or excrescence to a large cystic mass up to 8 cm in diameter. The most common site is the posterior wall in the region of the trigone. The surface of both large and small areas of endometriosis is characterized by irregular areas of bluish-gray or bluish-black discoloration covered by an intact vesical mucosa. A palpable bladder mass is present in the suprapubic area or vaginally in about 40% of cases. The mass is usually firm and slightly irregular and may be tender. During menstruation the areas of endometriosis appear to be larger, more congested, and of a deeper bluish-black color than otherwise. After removal or irradiation of the ovaries, the areas of endometriosis undergo progressive reduction in size and eventually disappear.

Histologically, the lesions are characterized by endometrial glands of varying size and shape scattered through the thickness of the bladder wall. The glands are lined by high or low columnar epithelium that are occasionally ciliated. The glands may be distended with blood or filled with necrotic material reflecting the various phases of the menstrual cycle in the same manner as does normally situated endometrium. The glands are surrounded by varying amounts of highly cellular endometrial stroma.

The symptoms of endometriosis of the bladder are correlated with the size and location of the lesion and the cyclic changes induced by ovarian hormonal activity. The most common and almost constant symptom is vesical discomfort, which is characterized by a sense of pressure, heaviness, cramping, or pain in the region of the bladder. The discomfort is most frequently noted in the suprapubic area and less commonly in the vesicovaginal area and rarely in the lumbar, perineal, or sciatic area. Urinary symptoms such as urgency, burning, frequency, dysuria, and tenesmus are found in the majority of cases. Gross hematuria is found in about 25% of cases.

The mechanism by which the displaced endometrium reaches the interior of the bladder is still disputed. Some believe it invades the bladder by direct extension or via lymphatics or blood vessels. Others believe that it is the result of growth of embryonic endometrial remnants in the bladder wall. Injury to the bladder at the time of operation is another possibility, and the finding that previous gynecologic or abdominal operations have been reported in the majority of cases of endometriosis of the bladder is used to support this viewpoint. Others believe that endometriosis of the bladder may represent an example of the multipotentiality of the serosal epithelium covering portions of the bladder.

AMYLOIDOSIS

Amyloidosis (Figs. 11.9, 11.10) is characterized as homogeneous, eosinophilic, extracellular hyaline masses located between bundles of collagen and muscularis.

Amyloid is usually deposited in the submucosa and upper two-thirds of the muscularis. The masses give reactions for amyloid such as yellow-green birefringence under polarized light after staining with Congo red. It is often deposited in the media of small arteries. A chronic inflammatory component of lymphocytes and plasma cells is often present. A few foreign body giant cells may be present and the amyloid may be focally calcified.

Amyloidosis is often classified into 2 groups:

1. Primary amyloidosis, which is not associated with any predisposing disease. Primary amyloidosis may occur in a generalized or localized form.

2. Secondary amyloidosis, which is associated with a recognized predisposing disease such as rheumatoid arthritis and chronic osteomyelitis or with neoplasms such as myeloma. Secondary amyloidosis is most often in the generalized form.

In most organs of the body, amyloidosis occurs as a generalized form as a manifestation of an underlying plasma cell neoplasm (myeloma) or plasmacytic dyscrasia. In the bladder, however, most cases of amyloidosis occur as a solitary, localized process.

Most observers have described the cystoscopic appearance of amyloidosis of the bladder as similar to that of an infiltrating neoplasm. In the majority of cases, a diagnosis of malignant tumor is entertained preoperatively. The lesions have varied from hemorrhagic ulcers to inflammatory-looking excrescences. Any portion of the bladder may be involved, and there may be multiple areas of bladder involvement. The bladder wall often appears thickened and has a nodular "cobblestone" appearance.

Less than 10% of patients with amyloidosis of the bladder will die of systemic amyloidosis. Therefore, the presence of an amyloid tumor in the bladder should not be necessarily regarded as a manifestation of myeloma. However, a thorough search for possible underlying disease should be initiated. If Bence-Jones proteinuria is absent, the serum electrophoretic pattern is normal, and if a rectal biopsy shows no evidence of amyloidosis, further evaluation is probably no longer necessary.

HEMANGIOMA

The bladder is an unusual site for a hemangioma (Figs. 11.11 to 11.14). The tumor is probably congenital and the increase in size with age is the result of enlargement of vascular channels as well as budding of new vessels. Hemangiomas of the bladder are slow growing tumors, which may explain why symptoms often develop in later years.

Grossly, hemangiomas vary in size from very small to massive lesions that may fill the entire lumen of the bladder. In a study of 40 hemangiomas, 17 were 3 cm or more in size, 12 were 1 to 3 cm, and 11 were less than 1 cm (10). The tumors are bluish in color, irregular in outline, sessile in structure, and soft in consistency. They may be found in any area of the bladder. The dome and trigone are the common sites. On cut section the tumors are well delimited but not encapsulated.

Microscopically, hemangiomas of the bladder are usually of the cavernous variety with large and small intercommunicating vascular spaces lined by a single layer of flat endothelial cells and filled with erythrocytes or serum. Atypicality of the endothelial lining cells is rarely observed. Many bladders develop numerous dilated vascular channels in the lamina propria. This is a normal variant of the vasculature of the bladder. These normal dilated vascular structures have abundant stroma between the vascular channels and do not present clinically as a tumor.

One-third to one-half of hemangiomas of the bladder are diagnosed under the age of 20. The remainder are diagnosed randomly at older ages. The sex incidence is equally distributed between male and female patients. The most common symptom is hematuria with repeated attacks over a long period. Size of the hemangioma may not correspond to the intensity or duration of bleeding. Other symptoms such as dysuria, frequency, urgency, acute renal retention, or renal colic may occur. About one-quarter of the cases have hemangiomas elsewhere in the body—usually centered around the labia, vagina, or penis.

Of 40 cases reported by Segal and Fink (10), only one was considered to be malignant. Smaller tumors can be fulgurated whereas larger ones must be removed through the suprapubic route. Following resection, recurrences have been noted in 10% to 20% of cases. When recurrences develop, it is probably due to incomplete removal of the tumor rather than to malignant change. Although hemangiomas of the bladder do not metastasize, direct extension to contiguous structures may take place.

PHEOCHROMOCYTOMA

Zimmerman et al. (11) first reported a case of pheochromocytoma (Figs. 11.15 to 11.18) of the urinary bladder in 1953. This patient complained of rapid heart beat after urination and at night when the bladder was full. These symptoms disappeared after removal of the tumor. While the etiology of pheochromocytoma of the bladder is not known, it is generally felt that the tumor arises from paraganglia related to the autonomic nerves of the bladder wall. This view is substantiated by studies by Copeland (12) who has shown that extra-adrenal paraganglia are widely dispersed in the human fetus. Although most of these paraganglia tissue disappear by the time adult life is reached, there is no valid reason why some parts of it may not persist as "rests" in such anomalous places as the bladder wall and occasionally give rise to tumor.

Pheochromocytomas are located within the muscular wall. They may occasionally be found incidentally on bladder biopsies performed for other reasons. However, about 80% of the tumors can be seen at cystoscopy. A wide range of tumor sizes occur.

The histological appearance of pheochromocytomas is the same as for pheochromocytomas in other sites. Rosenberg (13) in 1957, while reporting on the second known case of pheochromocytoma of the bladder, pointed out that "it is virtually impossible to determine pathologically whether a pheochromocytoma is benign or malignant since both types infiltrate locally and grow into blood vessels. The only sure way to diagnose a malignant pheochromocytoma is to find distant metastases in an area where pheochromocytomas are not expected to develop." Rosenberg's assessment still holds today.

The tumor may present at any age. The duration of symptoms in some cases suggests that the neoplasm may have been present since infancy. The sex distribution is approximately equal, and half of the patients will have hematuria. Typical symptoms are throbbing or pain in the head after micturation. Occasionally, patients have found that these symptoms are more severe when the bladder is full. The majority of patients have paroxysmal hypertension, a lesser number have sustained hypertension, and a few patients have no hypertension.

Almost all patients with paroxysmal hypertension become normotensive and asymptomatic following surgical removal of the tumor. Patients with sustained hypertension are less likely to become normotensive following surgical removal of the tumor. It has been stated that a persistently elevated excretion of urinary catecholamines after surgery means that a second tumor is present or there has been metastatic spread. However, one should not be misled by a high reading in the immediate postoperative period. Normal levels may not return for weeks or months after surgery. Why urinary catecholamines do not return to normal immediately after surgery has not been adequately explained. Ten to 20% of patients with bladder pheochromocytomas will have local recurrences and an equal number will have metastatic disease. The prognosis of these malignant tumors has been poor.

NEPHROGENIC ADENOMA (ADENOMATOID TUMORS)

In 1949 Davies (14) described a bladder hamartoma. From the description, this appears to be what today is termed "nephrogenic adenoma" or "adenomatoid tumor" (Figs. 11.19 to 11.22). In 1950 Friedman and Kuhlenbeck (15) found seven cases of similar tumors in the records of the Armed Forces Institute of Pathology.

These tumors were given the name "nephrogenic adenoma" because the initial observers were struck by the resemblance of these tumors to a renal tubular pattern. The tumors have a common feature of epithelial tubules lined by a single layer of cuboidal or columnar epithelium. Some of the tubules show cystlike dilatation. The tubules may be straight, looped, or convoluted and to some observers have a definite similarity to collecting tubules, loops of Henle, and distal convoluted tubules of the kidney. However, even those observers struck with this similarity admitted that the histology is not completely identical with kidney tubules. In retrospect, it appears that any similarity with renal structures is merely coincidental.

Nephrogenic adenomas present with hematuria in the majority of cases. Other symptoms include dysuria, frequency, nocturia, and discharge. These tumors may occur in any portion of the bladder mucosa. The trigone appears to be the most common location. They have variously been described as papillomatous, polypoid, or smooth glistening flattened tumors. The tumors have measured up to 7 cm.

The etiology of these lesions remains controversial. Possibilities include a response to chronic irritation, an expression of ectopic embryological remnants, or most likely, an expression of the diverse potentialities of bladder epithelium.

The vast majority of these tumors have followed a benign course. If not completely removed, they will recur. Several malignant nephrogenic adenomas have been reported (16). It is not entirely certain whether these malignant tumors were actually nephrogenic adenomas or other entities.

NEUROFIBROMAS

Neurofibromas (Figs. 11.23, 11.24) of the lower urinary tract are usually a manifestation of von Recklinghausen's disease. In a review of 25 cases, only seven were not associated with von Recklinghausen's disease (17).

Approximately one-third of the cases will occur in children whereas the majority of cases will be diagnosed in adult life. The trigone and the vesical neck are the most common sites of occurrence. Symptoms include frequency, abdominal pain, and obstruction. The symptoms may be nonspecific and very troublesome.

Neurofibromas can be distributed throughout the bladder as multiple nodules, a solitary mass, or diffuse thickening. Microscopic examination reveals a tumor composed of interweaving bundles of spindle-shaped cells with elongated nuclei. There generally is a poorly defined cytoplasm with varying degrees of myxoid stroma. The nuclei show a tendency to palisade and may be moderately enlarged and show considerable hyperchromasia.

Neurofibromas are capable of undergoing malignant transformation. Approximately 10% of neurofibromas of the bladder are given a diagnosis of malignancy. Metastases occur in only a few of these histologically malignant tumors. Because of the association with generalized symptoms, neurofibromatosis of the bladder should be considered in any patient with urinary tract symptoms who has cutaneous evidence or a familial history suggestive of the disorder.

ADDITIONAL BENIGN TUMORS

Lipomas, leiomyomas, fibromas, granular cell myoblastomas, fibromyxomas, myxomas, and dermoids have been reported in the urinary bladder. These tumors vary in size, clinical symptoms, and location in the bladder. They have the same histological features as their counterparts elsewhere. Malignant transformation is extremely rare.

REFERENCES

1. Packham, D. A. (1971): The epithelial lining of the female trigone and urethra. *Br. J. Urol.*, 43:201–204.
2. Koss, L. G. (1979): Mapping of the urinary bladder: its impact on the concepts of bladder cancer. *Hum. Pathol.*, 10:533–548.
3. Dimmette, R. M., Sproat, H. F., and Sayegh, E. S. (1956): The classification of carcinoma of the urinary bladder associated with schistosomiasis and metaplasia. *J. Urol.*, 75:680–686.
4. Holley, P. S., and Mellinger, G. T. (1961): Leukoplakia of the bladder and carcinoma. *J. Urol.*, 86:235–241.
5. Kelalis, P. P., Emmett, J. L., and DeWeerd, J. H. (1963): Leukoplakia of the urinary bladder: report of a case with unusual features. *Proc. Mayo Clin.*, 38:514–518.
6. O'Flynn, J. D., and Mullaney, J. (1967): Leukoplakia of the bladder. *Br. J. Urol.*, 39:461–471.
7. Judd, E. S. (1921): Adenomyomata presenting as tumor of the bladder. *Surg. Clin. North Am.*, 1:1271–1276.
8. Ball, T. L., and Platt, N. A. (1962): Urologic complications of endometriosis. *Am. J. Obstet. Gynecol.*, 84:1516–1520.
9. Abeshouse, B. S., and Abeshouse, G. (1960): Endometriosis of the urinary tract: a review of the literature and a report of 4 cases of vesical endometriosis. *J. Int. Coll. Surg.*, 34:43–62.
10. Segal, A. D., and Fink, H. (1942): Cavernous hemangioma, report of a case and review of literature. *J. Urol.*, 47:453–460.

11. Zimmerman, I. J., Biron, R. E., and MacMahan, H. E. (1953): Pheochromocytoma of the urinary bladder. *N. Engl. J. Med.*, 249:25–26.
12. Copeland, R. E. (1952): Prenatal development of abdominal para-aortic bodies in man. *J. Anat.*, 86:357–372.
13. Rosenberg, L. M. (1957): Pheochromocytoma of the urinary bladder. *N. Engl. J. Med.*, 257:1212–1215.
14. Davies, T. A. (1949): Hamartoma of the urinary bladder. *Northwest Med.*, 48:182–185.
15. Friedman, N. B., and Kuhlenbeck, H. (1950): Adenomatoid tumors of the bladder reproducing renal structures (nephrogenic adenomas). *J. Urol.*, 64:657–670.
16. Christoffersen, J., and Moller, J. E. (1972): Adenomatoid tumors of the urinary bladder. *Scand. J. Urol. Nephrol.*, 6:295–298.
17. Gonzalez-Angulo, A., and Reyes, H. A. (1963): Neurofibromatosis involving the lower urinary tract. *J. Urol.*, 89:804–811.

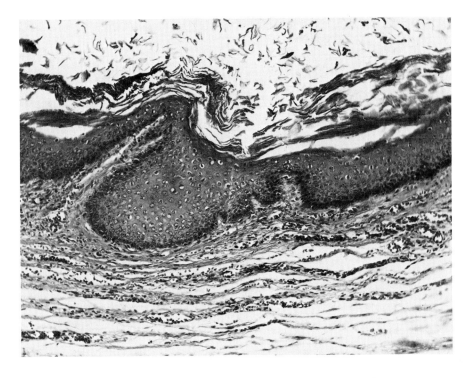

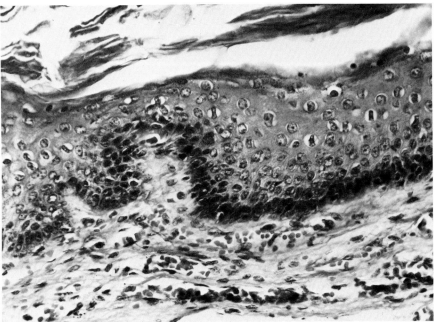

FIGS. 11.1, 11.2. Squamous metaplasia. ($\times$100 and $\times$200)

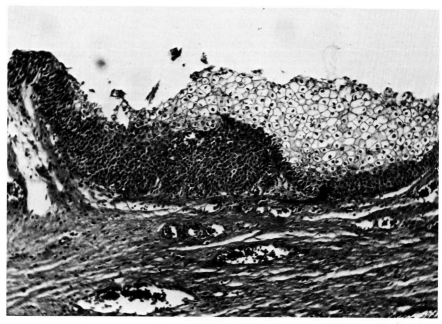

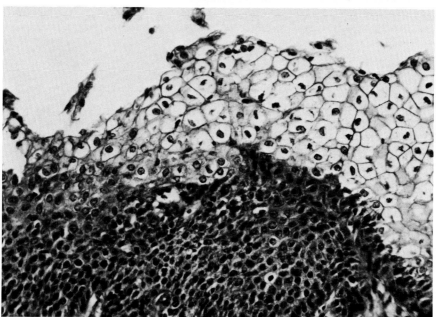

FIGS. 11.3, 11.4. Squamous metaplasia. (× 100 and × 200)

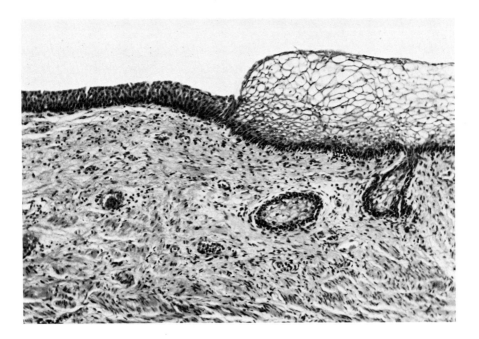

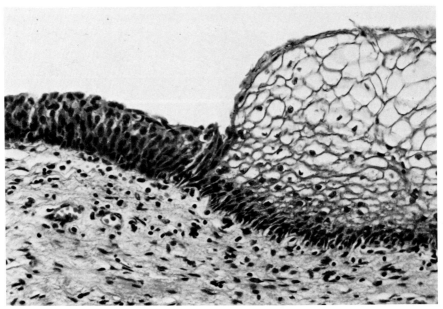

FIGS. 11.5, 11.6. Squamous metaplasia. ($\times$100 and $\times$200)

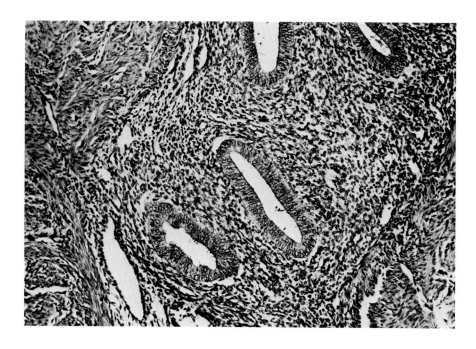

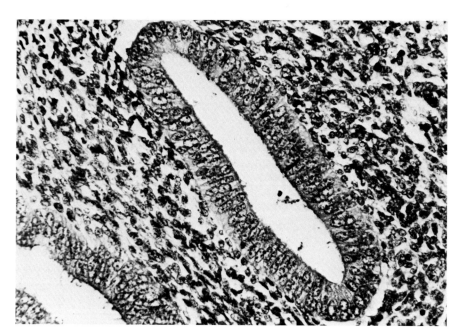

FIGS. 11.7, 11.8. Endometriosis of bladder. ($\times$100 and $\times$200)

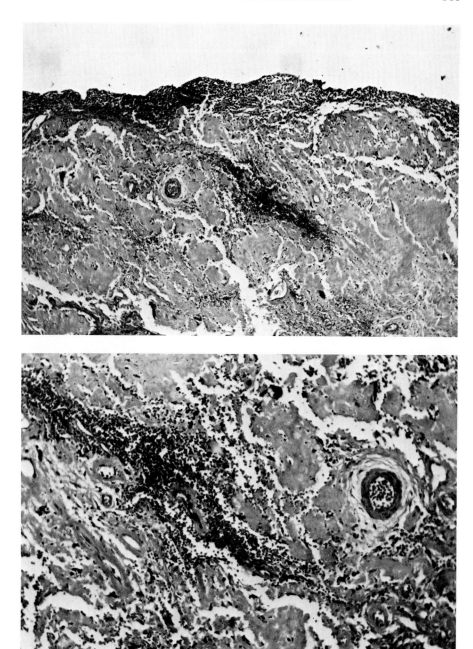

FIGS. 11.9, 11.10. Amyloidosis of bladder. ($\times$100 and $\times$200)

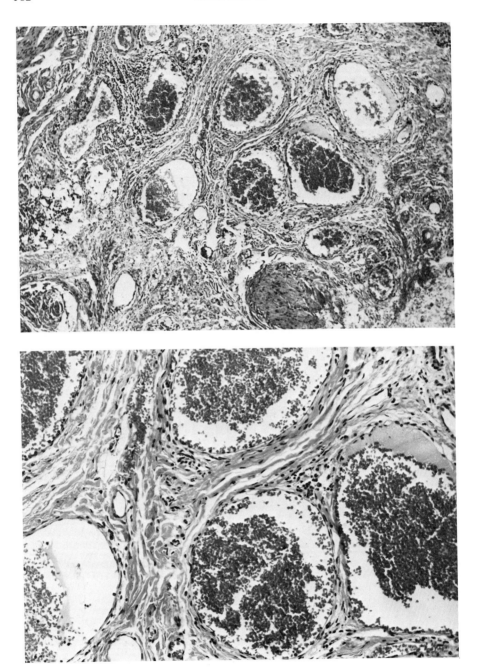

FIGS. 11.11, 11.12. Dilatation of normal vasculature of bladder. (×100 and ×200)

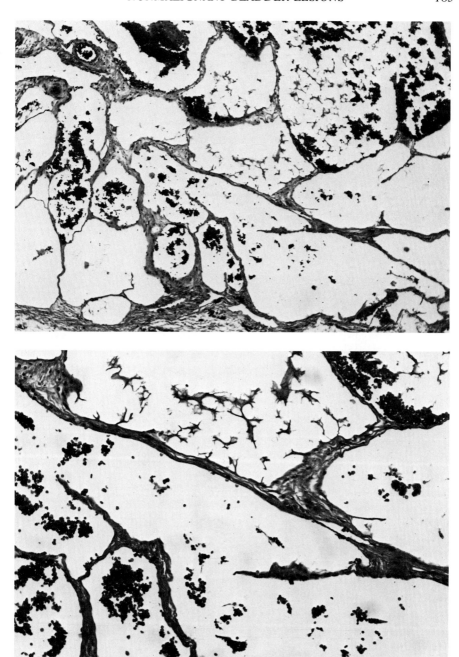

FIGS. 11.13, 11.14. Hemangioma of bladder. ($\times$100 and $\times$200)

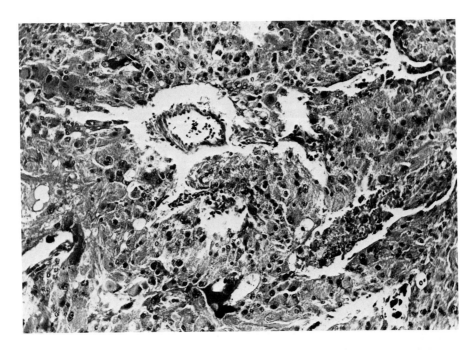

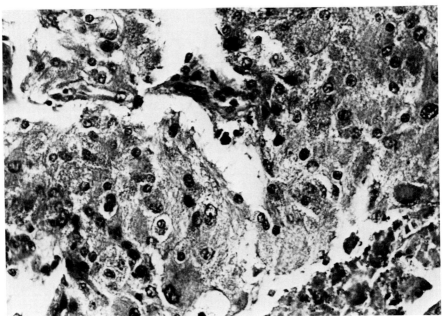

FIGS. 11.15, 11.16. Pheochromocytoma of bladder. (×100 and ×200)

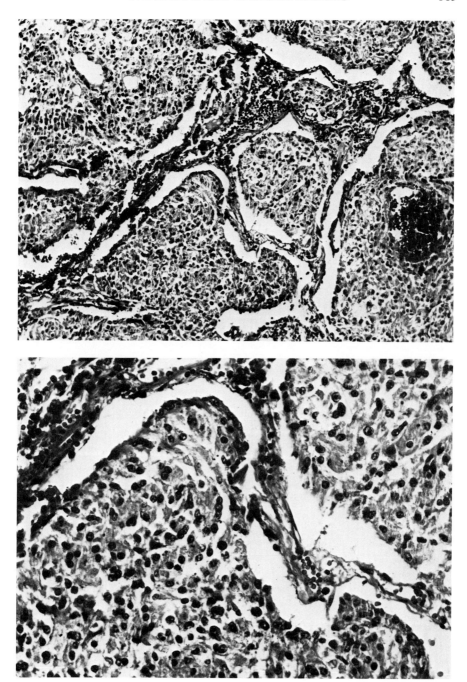

FIGS. 11.17, 11.18. Pheochromocytoma of bladder. ($\times$100 and $\times$200)

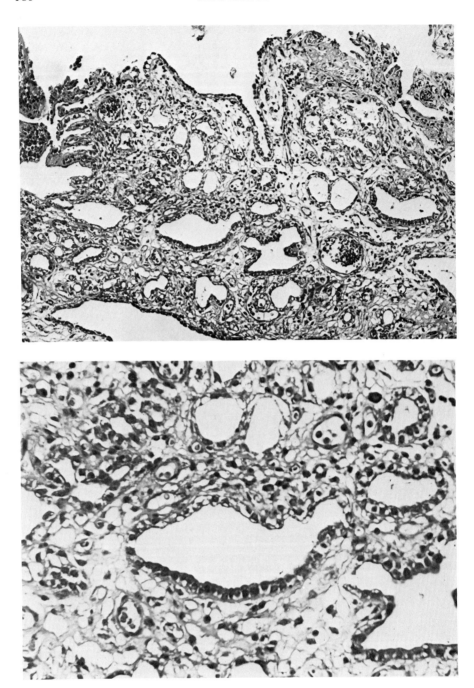

FIGS. 11.19, 11.20. Nephrogenic adenoma of bladder. (×100 and ×200)

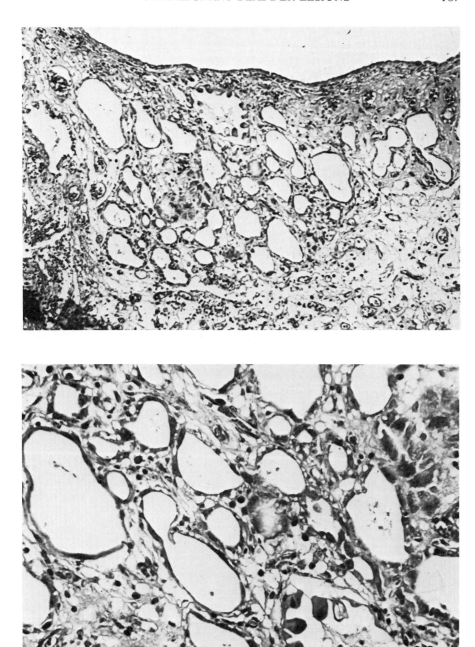

FIGS. 11.21, 11.22. Nephrogenic adenoma of bladder. ($\times$100 and $\times$200)

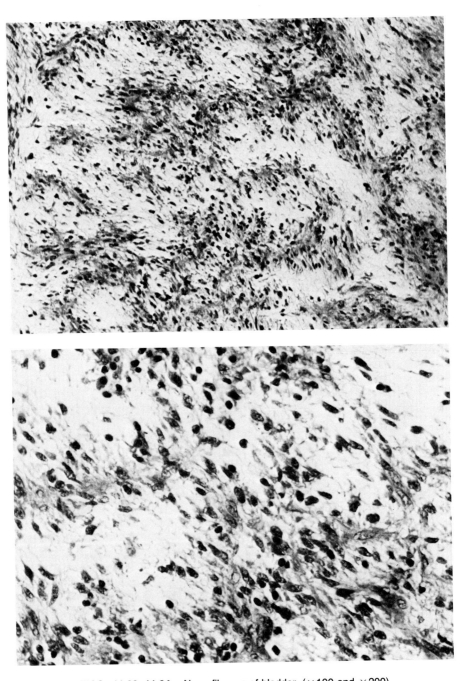

FIGS. 11.23, 11.24. Neurofibroma of bladder. (×100 and ×200)

Chapter 12

Miscellaneous Malignant Bladder Lesions

SARCOMA BOTRYOIDES

Crosse in 1830-1835, Staneley-Savoy in 1852, and Brickett in 1857 each described polyposis of the bladder in children (1). All three children died in a short time. Although microscopic proof is lacking, the gross descriptions appear to be similar to sarcoma botryoides (Figs. 12.1 to 12.10). The earliest reported case of sarcoma botryoides confirmed by microscopic examination is that of Monckberg in 1907 (2).

Grossly, the bladder shows multiple, soft, myxomatous, polypoid growths arising from the bladder mucosa. These growths have been characterized as having the appearance of a bunch of grapes or as closely resembling the gross structure of a hydatiform mole. The surface is usually smooth, shiny, and occasionally may have areas of ulceration. On cut section the tumor usually has a fleshy, firm homogeneous texture that is gray-white or gray-pink in color. Although any portion of the bladder may be affected, the growths arise near the trigone in approximately one-half the cases.

Sarcoma botryoides is considered to be a form of rhadomyosarcoma. The pathognomonic cells are immature and mature striated muscle fibers showing definite myofibrillae with or without cross striations. The general pattern is that of a loose-textured neoplasm with focal areas of hypercellularity and compactness. The latter is best seen immediately beneath the urothelium in the so-called "cambium" layer. Houette (3) described three types of cells characteristic of sarcoma botryoides. The first type of cell is rounded and slightly oval and about the size of a lymphocyte. However, the nucleus is lighter staining, and its chromatin network is more clearly seen than in a lymphocyte. The cytoplasm is eosinophilic and scanty. Occasional mitotic figures may be present. The second type of cell is elongated with a centrally placed nucleus and peripheral longitudinal fibrillae. The nuclei are hyperchromatic and contain a large amount of chromatin material and multiple nucleoli. In some fibers the nuclei are at the periphery of the fibers, and cross striations are seen in the cytoplasm. The third type of cell is a multinucleated giant cell containing numerous centrally located nuclei. Immediately surrounding the nuclei, the cytoplasm is densely eosinophilic whereas the periphery of the cytoplasm may show vacuolization.

It should be emphasized that the histological appearance of sarcoma botryoides changes with time. Early in the course of the disease, the predominant cell may be polymorphonuclear leukocytes, lymphocytes, and monocytes intermixed with occasional malignant cells in a myxomatous stroma. Some of the malignant spindle cells may show cross striations. In later stages of the disease, the three cells described by Houette become more apparent.

The majority of cases occur in childhood although cases have been described in elderly patients. The most common initial symptom is dysuria. Subsequent symptoms are related to inflammation and obstruction. Hematuria has been observed in a minority of cases.

The prognosis of sarcoma botryoides in the past has been dismal, with death usually occurring within 24 months of diagnosis. The causes of death were, in the majority of cases, debility produced by the tumor and ascending urinary infection caused by obstruction. Metastases to regional lymph nodes are rare. With more aggressive initial therapy, prognosis may improve in the future.

ADDITIONAL SARCOMAS

Primary sarcoma of the bladder accounts for less than 1% of all bladder malignancies (Figs. 12.11, 12.12). The symptoms depend on the location of the tumors, the rapidity of their growth, and the presence or absence of infection. Symptoms of bladder obstruction may result from involvement of the vesical neck or reduction of elasticity or capacity from generalized infiltration of the bladder wall. Renal failure may result from obstruction of the ureters. Infection is prone to develop early.

Diagnosis by cystoscopy is rare since the tumor begins in the deeper tissue involves the mucosa of the bladder late or not at all. In the early stages, the tumor is small, single, and fairly well localized. Growth may develop in one of two directions: (a) infiltration of the entire bladder wall with extension into the surrounding tissues without breaking through the bladder mucosa, and (b) growth toward the lumen in a bulky mass, reducing the capacity of the bladder. These tumors may erode through the bladder mucosa or cause a reactive proliferation of the overlying epithelium, which simulates a polypoid growth. The most common identifiable area of origin of sarcomas of the bladder is the trigone but in the majority of cases, the tumor is too far advanced to permit recognition of the area from which it has arisen.

Most primary sarcomas of the bladder have been described as fibrosarcoma, myosarcoma, or rhabdomyosarcoma (see the section Sarcoma Botryoides). The tumors are often composed of sarcoma cells that have bizarre, hyperchromatic, multinucleated cells with variable numbers of mitoses. Hemorrhage and necrosis may be present. A number of supposed sarcomas of the bladder have on review been reclassified as spindle cell carcinomas.

Primary sarcoma of the bladder infiltrates seminal vesicles, prostate, and rectum in males. In the female the uterus and adnexae are often involved. Metastases to the skull, skin, pleura, lungs, intestinal mucosa, liver, heart, and regional and inguinal lymph nodes have been reported. The overall prognosis of bladder sarcoma is poor. The average patient has survived less than a year after diagnosis.

OSSEOUS AND CARTILAGINOUS TUMORS

Osseous and cartilaginous tumors (Figs. 12.13, 12.14) are rare malignancies of the bladder. Ordonez (4) in 1856 reported the first case of a cartilage-containing tumor of the bladder. These tumors usually occur in middle-aged to elderly patients, and fall into two main categories—one where the bone and cartilage are neoplastic and the other where they are the result of metaplasia. The neoplastic tumors have metastasized, but in general they have followed a less malignant course than undifferentiated bladder sarcomas and primary osteosarcomas of bone.

LYMPHOMAS

Primary malignant lymphoma of the bladder (Figs. 12.15, 12.16) was first reported by Eve and then by Caffey, both in 1885 (5). The lesions remain a rarity today with secondary involvement from generalized lymphoma, most commonly lymphomas originating in the pelvis, being a more common event.

Primary lymphoma of the bladder is a disease of the middle-aged and elderly and appears to be more common in females. Intermittent hematuria, frequency of urination, and dysuria are the usual symptoms.

Grossly, the lesions may be solitary or have multiple growths. The growths may be smooth, rounded, or sessile, and are often covered with relatively normal mucosa. Most of the lesions are intramural, and ulceration is generally minimal.

A variety of terminology has been used to describe primary lymphoma of the bladder. There is no clear consensus as to what type of primary lymphoma is most likely to involve the bladder.

Primary lymphomas of the bladder tend to remain localized for a considerable period of time, although they are capable of direct extension to contiguous organs or distant metastases. Most observers have stressed the relatively favorable prognosis of primary lymphoma of the bladder as compared to lymphomas elsewhere.

METASTASES AND DIRECT EXTENSION TO THE BLADDER

The bladder is rarely the sole site of metastatic disease from a distant organ (Figs. 12.17 to 12.22). However, with disseminated malignancy, the bladder is not infrequently involved. In a Veterans Administration study of 5,200 autopsies, eight of 37 malignant melanomas, six of 125 gastric carcinomas, five of 688 lung carcinomas, and one of 96 pancreatic carcinomas metastasized to the bladder (6). In nonVeterans Administration patient populations, metastases from the breast are also seen. Presumably, any malignancy could conceivably metastasize to the bladder.

Direct extension from contiguous structures such as the colon, prostate, and cervix, or from lymphomas originating in the pelvis may occur. It is often difficult to determine with certainty whether bladder involvement in this setting is a result of direct extension of tumor or a result of metastases. Five to 10% of colon carcinomas will involve the bladder—usually the left lateral wall of the bladder. Carcinoma of the cervix or uterus usually involves the posterior bladder wall or floor in the midline.

Metastases from the kidney have been reported. Occasionally, it is difficult to determine whether these are metastases or represent reimplantation of exfoliated cells from the ureter/kidney or represent multifocal foci of tumor caused by unknown carcinogens affecting the entire urothelium.

Prostate carcinoma, in its inception, is a localized malignancy that rarely involves the bladder. However, those prostate carcinomas that increase in stage often directly extend into the bladder along the posterior urethra, bladder neck, or through the trigone. It is often difficult to distinguish with certainty prostate carcinomas extending into the bladder from invasive bladder carcinoma. Melicow (7) has shown that bone metastases from bladder carcinoma are not uncommon and "that in a patient with a tumor whose primary origin is in doubt (i.e., bladder versus prostate) the mere presence of radiographic evidence of bone involvement does not necessarily favor the prostate as the primary site." The clinical history plus acid phosphatase studies may be helpful in distinguishing these tumors.

ADDITIONAL MALIGNANT TUMORS

Signet ring carcinomas, carcinosarcomas, germ cell tumors such as choriocarcinoma and teratocarcinoma, and carcinoid tumors have been reported as primary malignancies of the bladder.

REFERENCES

1. Brickett, J. (1858–59): *Royal Med. Chir. Soc. (London)*, 41:311–321.
2. Monckberg, J. G. (1907): Uber heterotope mesodermale geschwulste am unteren ende der urogenitalapparates. *Virchows Arch. Pathol. Anat.*, 187:471–516.
3. Houette, C. (1929): Rhaodomyome diverticulaire congenital de la vessie. *Ann. Anat. Pathol. (Paris)*, 6:267–282.
4. Ordonez, M. E. C. (1856): *Gaz. Med. (Paris)*, 11:824.
5. Jacobs, A., and Symington, T. (1953): Primary lymphosarcoma of urinary bladder. *Br. J. Urol.*, 25:119–125.
6. Sheehan, E. E., Greenberg, S. D., and Scott, R. (1963): Metastatic neoplasms of the bladder. *J. Urol.*, 90:281–284.
7. Melicow, M. M. (1955): Tumors of the urinary bladder: a clinicopathological analysis of over 2500 specimens and biopsies. *J. Urol.*, 74:498–519.

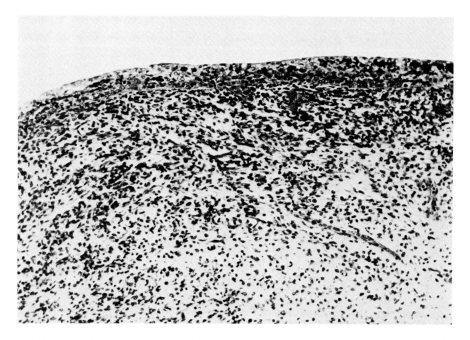

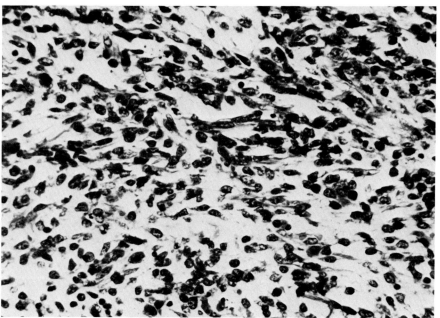

FIGS. 12.1, 12.2. Sarcoma botryoides. ($\times$100 and $\times$200)

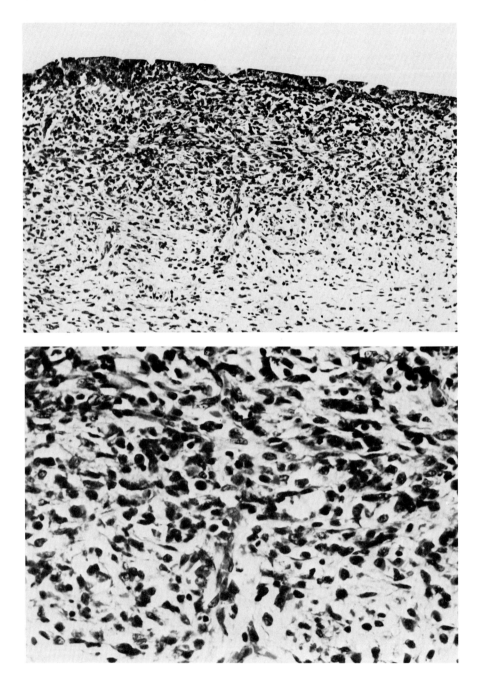

FIGS. 12.3, 12.4. Sarcoma botryoides. ($\times$100 and $\times$200)

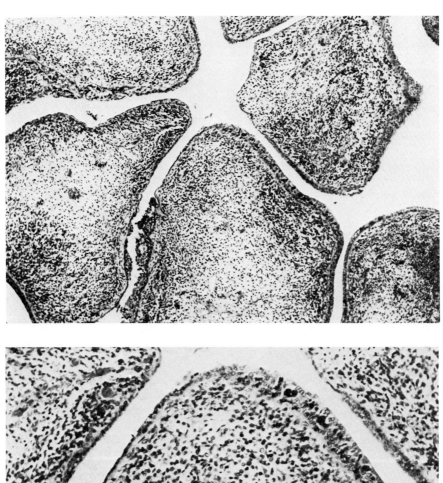

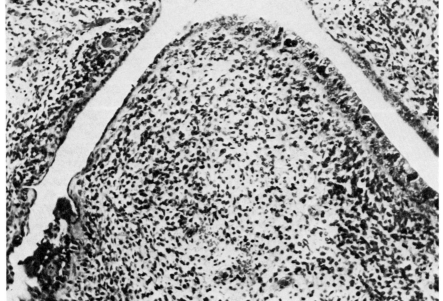

FIGS. 12.5, 12.6. Sarcoma botryoides. (×40 and ×100)

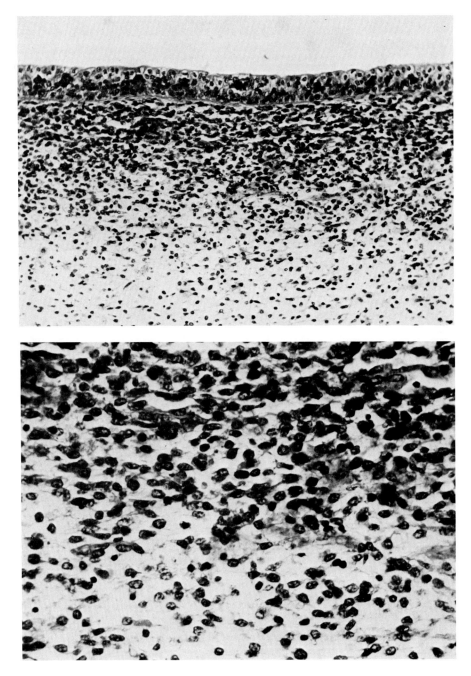

FIGS. 12.7, 12.8. Sarcoma botryoides. (×100 and ×200)

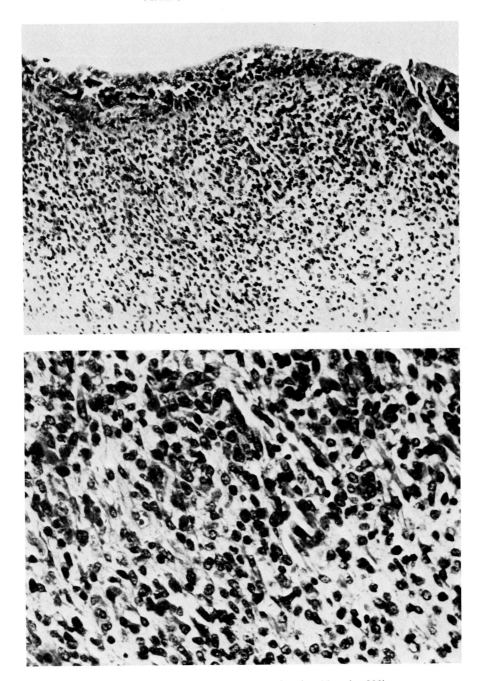

FIGS. 12.9, 12.10. Sarcoma botryoides. (×100 and ×200)

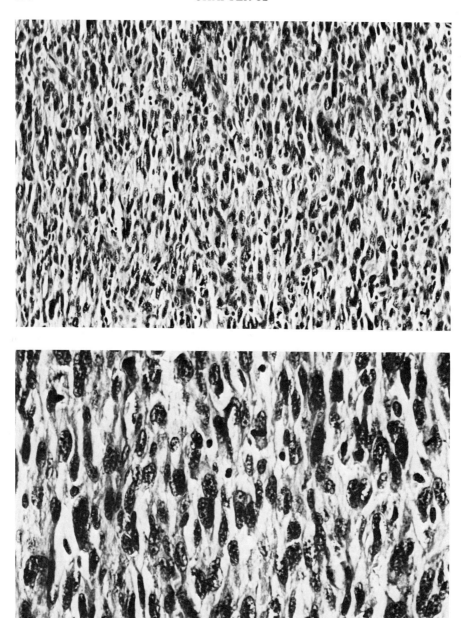

FIGS. 12.11, 12.12. Sarcoma of bladder. ($\times 100$ and $\times 200$)

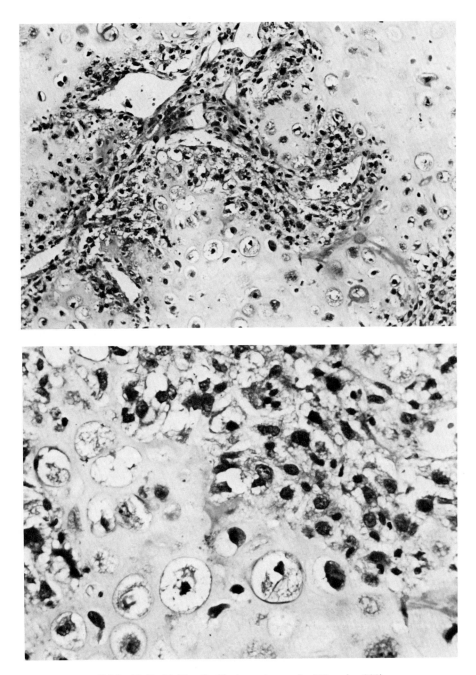

FIGS. 12.13, 12.14. Cartilaginous tumor. (×100 and ×200)

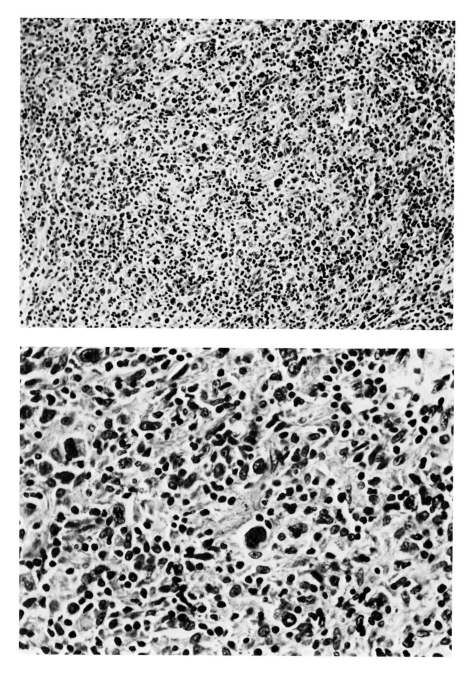

FIGS. 12.15, 12.16. Lymphoma of the bladder. (×100 and ×200)

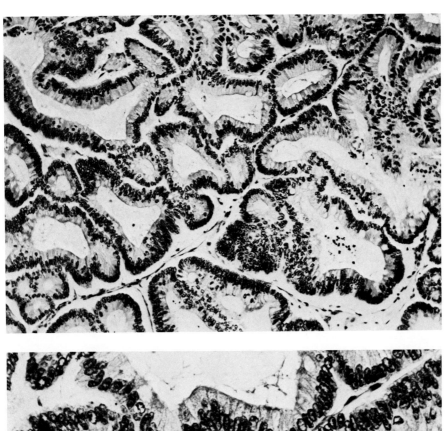

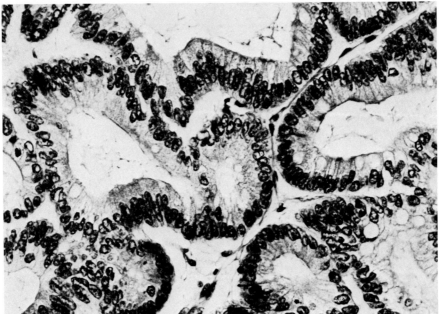

FIGS. 12.17, 12.18. Colon carcinoma involving the bladder. ($\times$100 and $\times$200)

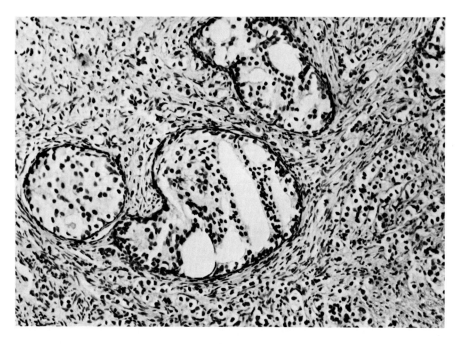

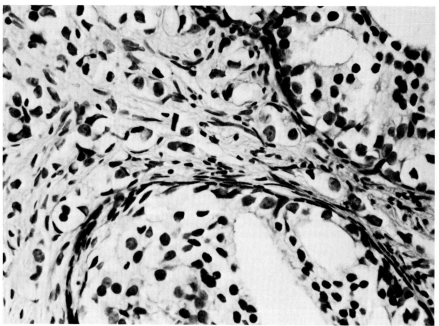

FIGS. 12.19, 12.20.   Prostate carcinoma involving the bladder. (×100 and ×200)

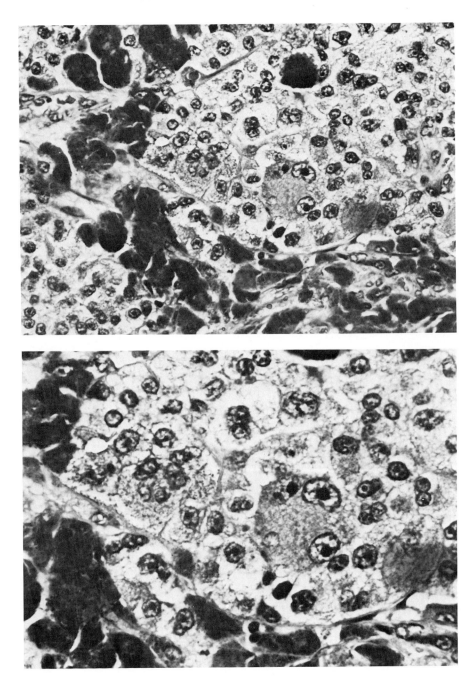

FIGS. 12.21, 12.22. Malignant melanoma involving the bladder. ($\times$ 100 and $\times$ 200)

Subject Index

Subject Index